THE ULTIMATE PRESCRIPTION

THE
ULTIMATE
PRESCRIPTION

What the Medical Profession Isn't Telling You

DR. JAMES L. MARCUM, MD
with CHARLES MILLS

Tyndale House Publishers, Inc.
CAROL STREAM, ILLINOIS

Visit Tyndale online at www.tyndale.com.

Visit Dr. Marcum's website at www.heartwiseministries.org.

TYNDALE and Tyndale's quill logo are registered trademarks of Tyndale House Publishers, Inc.

The Ultimate Prescription: What the Medical Profession Isn't Telling You

The Ultimate Prescription first published in 2011 by Tyndale House Publishers, Inc.

Designed by Ron Kaufmann

Edited by Susan Taylor

The names of the patients in this book have been changed to protect their privacy.

Library of Congress Cataloging-in-Publication Data

Marcum, James.
   The ultimate prescription : what the medical profession isn't telling you / James L. Marcum with Charles Mills.
     p. cm.
   Rev. ed. of: The heart of health.
   ISBN 978-1-4143-6817-7 (sc)
1. Health—Religious aspects—Christianity. 2. Medicine—Religious aspects—Christianity. I. Mills, Charles, 1950- II. Marcum, James. Heart of health. III. Title.
   BT732.M32 2011
   261.5'61—dc23
                                     2011040453

Printed in the United States of America

17   16   15
7   6   5   4

I would like to dedicate this book to my parents,
Jim and Mary Marcum,
who have taught and supported me throughout my life.
They have focused my learning
on what the Great Physician teaches.
This book exists because of their love and guidance.

Contents

ACKNOWLEDGMENTS

THERE ARE SO MANY who have contributed to this project. I hope they realize how important they are to me. Charles Mills is more than a "with." He has been a friend, a mentor, and a gigantic creative force. He has brought together ideas given to me by the Holy Spirit and merged them with the insights shared by the many healers he has interviewed through the years.

Dorinda Mills is always there supporting and contributing to Charles's ministry.

To Jeannie Hart, Michelle Rapkin, Nena Madonia, and the staff at Right Time Right Place: your guidance, belief in the project, and counsel during this process have been invaluable.

The people at Tyndale House, including John Farrar, Susan Taylor, Kara Leonino, Christy Wong Stroud, and Ron Kaufmann, have been vital to presenting the message of this book to the world.

I could not have completed this project without the support of my wife, Sonya, and my children, Kelli and Jake. I love you.

A special note of appreciation to my nurses, Lara and Kathy, who allow me to be so efficient with my time. Arvid and Doreen Jacobson always seem to offer the right words of encouragement.

To my patients and friends who have helped this project become a reality: I thank you for blessing my life during the twenty-year journey.

Finally, I want to publicly offer special thanks and praise to God, who has guided this book all along through the Holy Spirit, bringing together a team to take this message to the world. To Him all glory be given. I am so grateful for His enduring love and patience.

INTRODUCTION

At this very moment, you and I are part of the largest, most comprehensive health study this world has ever known. It's not being funded by a well-respected organization like the National Institutes of Health or the American Medical Association. There are no highly trained scientists bending low over colorful test tubes or peering pensively into microscopes, searching for clues. No forms are being filled out or random samples being taken. This study is quietly, unobtrusively being carried out in our homes, our schools, and our places of business.

The goal of this far-reaching investigation is to answer three simple questions. The first is, *What happens to the human body when it does everything . . . wrong?* What happens when it continues to take in toxic, nutritionally deficient foods, gets less than the necessary amount of sleep, is deprived of sufficient water intake, is inundated with a steady stream of harsh chemicals, is introduced to a never-ending supply of devastating, side-effect-laden pharmaceuticals, and is forced to breathe a constant flow of polluted air?

The second question is similar to the first, but it has to do with the human mind: *What happens when the information pouring into a brain's neural network is wrong?* What happens when it's taught to focus entirely on its own needs, its own desires, and its own happiness, at the expense of all else?

Finally, the study is examining people's spiritual lives, asking the third question: *What happens to a person's relationship with God when that relationship is based on beliefs that are built on flawed foundations, on images of God that are totally, heartbreakingly wrong?*

The results are pouring in. We can see them at the mall, on television, on the Internet, and in line at the bank. We can catch glimpses of them as we talk with coworkers or even strangers on the street, when we read the blogs of "experts" on the web, and when we scan the evening news sources. We can see them at our local churches, in the halls of Congress, and especially in crowded doctors' offices.

Many of us see the results of this ongoing study reflected back to us from our own mirrors. We find ourselves gazing into the faces of overweight, overworked, overstimulated people we hardly recognize. We lean forward and squint into the eyes of people who haven't a clue about what's going on inside our own bodies, yet we know that all isn't right in there—that something bad is happening deep inside us. We understand—although we don't know how or why—that something important is missing, something necessary for the days, weeks, and years ahead. But all we can do is stand there, unsure, confused, and afraid.

That's what happens when the human body, mind, and spirit become so wrapped up with what tastes good, feels good, and seems good that we lose sight of what really *is* good. That's what happens when truth is hidden and people start to depend on a random set of highly polished, expertly marketed, and decidedly deadly . . . lies.

In the condition that civilization has placed itself, doctors don't know what to do beyond treating symptoms and hoping for the best. Psychiatrists shake their heads in disbelief, wondering how their patients could ever get so emotionally messed up when they have so much for which to live. Pastors gaze down from their pulpits at dwindling flocks, searching for a way to transform what seems to have become an unattractive, seemingly inattentive, and reportedly highly agitated God into someone worth worshiping. And while parents juggle their overstretched budgets to cover astronomical medical insurance premiums and the costs of a growing list of prescription drugs, they must stand helplessly by as their children are attacked by diseases that used to afflict only the elderly.

Very Different

Life hasn't always been this way. One hundred years ago, the world was a very different place, filled with people living very different lives. The vast majority of people lived in the rural countryside, and in America, many lived on family farms. Most families grew and ate their own food. They didn't eat food marketed to them by national corporations that commercially processed their nourishment with heavy amounts of fats, salt, and added calories.

Social life was centered around the family unit, and the local church was the hub of activity in a community. A majority of the populace enjoyed a weekly day of rest, and the Bible was often the most read book in the home. Physical activity? That went hand in hand with what it took to survive or simply to put food on the table. They walked places instead of rode, drank water instead of pop, went to bed with the sun instead of after the late news, and found pleasure in creative—not passive—outlets. As a result of their rural lifestyle, people were less likely to suffer from the conditions so prevalent today; obesity, diabetes, heart disease, and many forms of cancers were not the mainstay of the medical literature and the media of the day. Sure the technology was not as advanced in detection, but these conditions of excess just were not described.

All that has changed. Today, we tend to eat whatever is convenient, dumping copious amounts of highly processed foods down our throats and hardly ever glancing at nutrition labels. Our cuisine is saturated with chemicals placed there to preserve "freshness" and turn us into addicts who will keep coming back for more. Television commercials scream their audio-enhanced messages urging overconsumption as families eat on the run, rarely sitting down to enjoy a healthy meal together.

We listen to the chirping of iPhones instead of birds. We spend more time indoors than out. We let the media define our thoughts, telling us what's important in life. Texting is replacing talking. Watching is replacing reading. Like sheep without a shepherd, we're allowing "media darlings" and other random strangers to dictate our thoughts and agendas. We're overmedicated and undernourished. The family unit is eroding, and God is becoming less and less important in our lives. When we finally exhaust ourselves in our constant strain to have everything, all the time, increasing numbers of us look around at our lives, judge them worthless, and decide life isn't worth living anymore. The rest of us simply stare into our mirrors and wonder why we're sick so much of the time.

The Good News

I have some good news for you, and you don't have to be a rocket scientist to understand it. We're in this tragic condition because we weren't designed to live life this way. It's as simple as that. The One who made us, who lovingly formed us from the "dust of the ground" according to Genesis 2:7, had a very different lifestyle in mind. We were designed to live in harmony with nature, not to manipulate it to our liking or financial gain. We were created to live a life free of undue stress, not to run ourselves 24/7, as if doing anything less were unacceptable. We were supposed to be creative creatures, not passive couch potatoes who spend our lives being entertained by the creative efforts of others. Most important, we were designed to worship the God who made us, not spend our lives running away from Him.

In short, we were designed to worship our Creator, love one another, and care for the earth. The further we distance ourselves from that ideal, the sicker we become.

Where Do I Start?

When I sat down to write this book, I was almost overwhelmed by the challenges ahead. Where would I start? What would be the very first words? How could I bring to the world a plan of action that would make a real difference in people's lives, that would change people, that would literally save them from years of disease and suffering? Should I use a scientific approach and find double-blind, randomized, placebo-controlled trials to prove and promote the truths found in the original human "owner's manual," the Bible? The scientific community would certainly appreciate that approach. Should I compile all the great works of God's healers throughout time and weave them into one gigantic volume? The literary community would be thrilled.

But in the quiet of soul-searching contemplation, I felt God asking me to write about the things I have seen and heard over the years as a cardiologist. I want this book to be personal—me talking to you about what I've discovered to be at the very heart of good health. I want to share with you, not only doctor-to-patient but friend-to-friend, the many deceptions that cloud our lives and make us sick.

Am I qualified to do this? Why should you want to read a book by James Marcum? What makes me so special? The answer lies not in the messenger but in the message. The power of this book doesn't lie in the words and studies and nutritional information you'll read. It's not dependent on the depth of research conducted or the degrees held by people I've quoted. The power of this book is entirely dependent on the work of the Holy Spirit, both in its writing and in its reading.

The truth is, I "practice" the healing arts. But God *created* them. And it is to God that I want to refer you and every patient who comes to see me, because He is what's missing in the lives of so many people. He holds the answer to every illness, every condition, and every heartbreak. He is the "Great Physician," the only true healer, the One who can touch lives and make us whole again.

That's why I've written this book. Because I believe God has given me a message to share with you.

In the pages that follow, I plan to introduce you to some of my patients and talk about how the very questions you're asking about your health are being answered in their lives.

Most Influential

I was reading about a recent poll of men who were asked who they thought was the most influential man today. This would be the individual to whom they looked for answers, someone they wanted to emulate.

Number one on the list was Don Draper, a character on the television series *Mad Men*. He's not even a real person!

Number two was Usain Bolt, an Olympic gold medalist who, many believe, defines the true spirit of competition.

President Barack Obama slipped in as number three.

While this poll may or may not reflect the feelings of most men, it was just another example of how the media have the power to create an influential character, market him as an ideal to the world, and influence the minds of a large segment of the population. The media are doing this same thing when it comes to telling us how to build and maintain optimum health. They're busily promoting dangerous medications, toxic foods, destructive lifestyles, and dubious cures. All this leads us to the question, who controls the media? Who, or *what*, is pulling the strings on the most powerful influence in our world today?

As for the poll I talked about previously, wouldn't it be nice if the person listed as the most influential man in this world were the man who loves us most; who provides true answers to life's troubling questions; who is, right at this moment, bending beside you as you read this book? Wouldn't it be nice if the one who received the most votes had been the One who longs to hold you in His arms, remembers the day you were born, appreciates the good in you, wants to eradicate the bad, and is building a future for you that exceeds your wildest dreams? Why didn't He make the top-ten list?

The reason is that the deceptions under which we're all living include not only what God does but what He *is*.

I want to tell the world that He's number one in my life. And I want you to know that the answers you're looking for when it comes to physical, mental, and spiritual healing can be found in Him.

Are you ready to uncover these deceptions? Are you ready to find the truth in an error-filled world? Then let's begin our journey back to health through the discovery of the ultimate prescription.

—James Marcum, MD

1

A VICTIM OF DECEPTION

It was 2:00 a.m. on Wednesday when my pager went off. Tuesday is a "call night" for me, which means I'm available all night for any and all situations that need my attention at the hospital. I should have known better than to think I'd enjoy a full night's sleep.

The familiar number illuminated on my pager identified the source. I dialed it quickly, and the emergency room doctor picked up on the first ring. "We've got a male, thirty-eight years old, experiencing severe chest pains and heart arrhythmia. I'm thinking MI."

My colleague was right. The symptoms were common for myocardial infarctions. I knew the man in the emergency room was quickly running out of time and, if something wasn't done soon, he could die.

When I arrived in the exam room, "the patient" became David. He was now very real to me—a man with pale skin and terrified eyes. His blood pressure was dangerously low, he had already received a dose of aspirin to thin his blood, and he was hooked up to a beeping electrocardiogram (EKG) machine.

I introduced myself and quickly scanned his chart. This was serious. Very serious. After breathing a quick prayer on my patient's behalf, I began to explain to him that he needed a procedure to open up the artery supplying the front of his heart with blood and I was going to assemble a team to fly him by helicopter to a facility where this operation could take place.

What happened next took only a few moments, but it seemed to last forever. David slumped down onto the examination table as his heart rhythm became completely random and unstable. The condition caused the blood to stop circulating in his body—a condition called ventricular tachycardia. Within seconds, he had passed out completely.

A team of highly skilled caregivers rushed into the room. The skin on David's chest was uncovered, and two electrode pads were attached to a device called a defibrillator by wires. These pads were placed over his heart. A shock of electricity jolted his body, causing it to convulse slightly as all eyes turned to the EKG. Sure enough, the waves of lines indicating the patient's heartbeats ceased their wild and random dance and settled once again into a steady ba-*beat*, ba-*beat*, ba-*beat*. David's eyes fluttered open, and he stared up at me for a moment, unsure of what was going on.

"How do you feel?" I asked.

"I'm okay," he responded weakly, glancing about at the other faces in the room, wondering where all those people had come from.

When I asked him about his pain, he said it was gone. I noticed that his blood pressure and heart rhythm had normalized, and for the moment, at least, my patient was out of danger. David had been dying and had been pulled back into life using a now-common technology. I whispered a prayer of thanks to the God who taught medical professionals how to perform "miracles" using the simple tools found in most modern hospitals.

As preparations for David's flight to the operating facility continued, I walked into the waiting room to talk with David's wife and two daughters. They had heard the alarms. They'd seen the technicians running down the hallway. They knew that something was very wrong with their husband and daddy. And they were terrified. Panic showed in their eyes as they desperately clung to one another, trying to maintain a grip on sanity.

"How could this happen?" David's wife wanted to know after I had explained the situation. "He's never been sick a day in his life!"

How Could This Happen?

How could this happen? I hear that question often. The answer isn't easy, and I told David's wife, Debbie, that I would explain everything as best I could later. But for now, we had to make sure that her husband was getting the acute care he needed.

David's left anterior descending coronary artery showed a 98 percent blockage. His heart simply was not receiving enough blood to function normally. The situation would be similar to having your air supply 98 percent blocked when you're trying to climb a mountain. That would affect not only your ability to breathe but also the ability of every organ in your body—including your heart—to function. Blood—pumped by the heart—carries oxygen up to the top of your head and down to the tips of your toes. In essence, when your heart stops functioning correctly, your entire body begins to suffocate.

Within minutes, a stent—a device to keep an artery open—was placed in David's coronary artery so blood could flow freely again. My patient was fortunate that no permanent damage to his heart or other organs had taken place during his sudden heart attack and dangerous rhythm on the examination table. I guess the best place to have a cardiac event is in a hospital while carrying on a conversation with a cardiologist!

This is where some well-meaning people miss an important point. We hear a lot about alternative medicines, potent herbal cures, or the importance of diet and exercise. And I will be the first to champion anything that has been proven to work. But there is, and always will be, a place for modern medicine, *especially* in emergency situations. If I have a heart attack, I want a stent. If my heart is going too slowly, give me a pacemaker. If I am bleeding to death, stop my bleeding and start a transfusion. If I have a bacterial infection, bring me some antibiotics. Without modern medicine, a whole lot of people would not be around to explore alternative medicines, examine herbal cures, or learn the importance of diet and exercise.

David was suffering an acute event brought on by a chronic condition. As I later dug into his history, I began to understand why he ended up on my examination table. His heart disease was caused by elements in his life bringing stress on his body. He smoked. He held a high-pressure job. He ate food practically devoid of nutrition. But did he, his wife, or his two precious daughters recognize those stressors as the cause of his heart disease? No. Because they, like many of us, were operating under some serious misconceptions, and no one was making the lifestyle connection for them.

As important as modern medicine and its technologies are, people fall victim to a number of misconceptions regarding what modern medicine can and can't do. We'll discuss these later in the book, but the first misconception is huge, so let's take a look at that one before we go any further.

The First Misconception

What is a misconception anyway? Doesn't it depend on a person's point of view or perception? Not really. It's a falsehood, a lie, a trick, or an untruth. These are all around us and have been almost since the beginning of time. Sometimes they are so elaborate that even the most astute people don't recognize the untruth. But 99 percent truth is still a lie. Good and intelligent people are being deceived or have become clueless concerning many of the facts of life. Why? Amazingly, the reason usually comes down to money.

More specifically, I want to suggest that the misconception exists because of selfishness. We—and the society in which we live—tend to put ourselves above the interests of others, often because of a desire for money, power, or control.

One current misconception is the idea that modern medicine can fix anything. But to be brutally honest, modern medicine can't *fix* a thing. What it can do is a pretty good job of dealing with the *symptoms* of a lot of things.

"But, Dr. Marcum," I can hear you say, "how about a broken leg? Doesn't a doctor fix that?"

It's true that the doctor can *set* the leg. He or she can make it so you don't have to limp for the rest of your life. But as for the healing of that broken bone, the doctor can only watch and be amazed.

"How about cancer?" you ask. "Don't we praise God for cancer survivors?"

Absolutely! But many others who receive the same treatment, experience the same therapy, go through the same procedures die of their disease. Regardless of the survival rate, nothing was fixed. At best we'd have to say that a rampaging cancer was slowed—which is a good thing indeed. Life was extended through the application of modern medicine. Unfortunately, that extension often comes at a terrible price, including mutilation and collateral damage to other organs.

And here's the scary part: people who have heart disease, who suffer from cancer, who fight debilitating pain, who stand in lines at drugstores waiting to fill their endless prescriptions, who sit and watch television commercials extolling the power of the latest and greatest pharmaceutical firmly believe that their doctors or the pills are providing a cure to their ills. They think they're getting "fixed." But the truth is, they're wrong.

So what do we do when we're facing a health crisis? The short answer is "It depends on the crisis." The long answer is "It depends on the cure."

I divide illness into two categories: acute illness and chronic illness. *Acute* means that something needs to be done right now, this second, or a patient could die. That certainly describes David as his heart malfunctioned on the examination table. He needed action, and he needed it now.

Chronic describes a condition of ongoing, frequent duration, one that is always present. Although David's heart attack was sudden and acute, it was the result of something that had been going on for a very long time. Arteries do not fill up with plaque overnight. That is why, when his wife asked, "How could this happen?" I knew I needed more information about my patient before I could answer her fully. David's heart attack wasn't the problem. It was the *result* of the problem.

Modern medical technology can be breathtaking in its effectiveness in treating acute illnesses. For instance, an article in the August 2011 issue of the medical journal *Circulation* reported that the average period from the time a patient arrives in the emergency room with a heart attack to the treatment to open the artery is down to sixty-four minutes. This is an amazing use of modern medicine to save lives every day. Most people are completely unaware of what goes on behind the closed doors of science laboratories and medical institutions. Our ability to learn and understand the universe and the human body is expanding faster than at any time in history. Force fields are no longer science fiction. Machines can now render objects invisible. Using atom smashers, scientists are hoping to discover more about the universe and the relationships between energy and matter. With enough energy, they are hoping to actually *create* matter. Teleportation of matter (the act of moving something simply by thought) is more than a theory at this point. Some discoveries are even being kept secret because of their military significance.

There are now computers performing unbelievable computations. Our DNA has been sequenced, providing a glimpse not only into what is but also into what may be. I've been reading about something called nanotechnology, in which scientists are making very, very small particles capable of going into cells, diagnosing a problem, and delivering specialized medicines to address that problem.

Yes, there is a place for technology. But this same body of knowledge is accomplishing something unexpected. Using these new devices and techniques, we are now discovering how activities such as worship can change chemical reactions in our bodies—reactions that affect every cell, muscle, and organ. We can identify how rest, nutrition, and even laughter help cure our ills and strengthen our immune systems. These "treatments" enable disease to be fought at the cellular level. This information has not been readily made available. And there's a reason, which we'll identify later.

But there's a downside to advancing technology. As it expands, we tend to look more and more at what *we* can do as human beings. We start worshiping at the altar of science instead of at the feet of the One who made us. As we start to see our symptoms diminish, we think we've found a cure. So who needs God? And the deception deepens.

The most important question we need to be asking ourselves is not, How can we get well? but rather, *Why are we sick?* That is the only question that can lead to finding the "ultimate fix."

Number One Killer

Cardiovascular disease is the number one killer in America, and its worldwide prevalence continues to rise. Some sources will contend that doctors, hospitals, medications, overdosages, and medical errors are surpassing cardiovascular disease as the number one source of death, and this may be true. But both statistics support the same conclusion. Neither patients nor doctors are clear about what exactly causes heart disease and how best to combat it. There are many theories regarding the causes.

One common theory blames inflammation and damage to the inner layer of blood vessels, the endothelium. Another theory is that the real cause of the condition is genetic. But genetic alterations take many, many generations to develop. Heart disease was practically unheard of a hundred years ago, and there are still places on earth where very few suffer from this condition. For instance, in Africa, rural China, and other parts of the world where the diet is less Western (in other words, more plant based), the prevalence of cardiovascular disease is much lower.

In about half the cases of cardiovascular disease, the first manifestation is a heart attack. In other words, patients don't know the attacks are coming, and their doctors are not entirely clear about what triggers the attacks. That is why education is crucial.

Over the next twenty-four hours, around three thousand American hearts will malfunction. This is nearly the same number of persons who died in the tragedy of September 11,

2001. This comes to 1.1 million heart attacks a year. One out of three people will die at the time of the initial event or within the first twelve months after it.

Forty percent of Americans have cardiovascular disease of some sort, and in women the death rate from this condition is eight times higher than the death rate from cancer. In fact, in women, cardiovascular disease poses a greater risk than breast cancer and all other diseases *combined*. Those numbers continue to climb.

I need to say something that may startle and even anger you. But I'm just the messenger, so please don't shoot. *It has been estimated that 80 to 90 percent of cardiovascular disease is acquired*. That's right. The painful truth is that we give the disease to ourselves by the choices we make over a lifetime. We create the chronic condition that brings about the acute event by placing endless stressors on our systems—stressors that eventually do us in.

David did not even know he had a problem until that early Wednesday morning when he felt as if an elephant had sat down on his chest to rest. I thank God that after the event, David began his search for the ultimate prescription. When he was faced with death, he started to evaluate the reasons he had a heart attack.

2

SEARCHING FOR TRUTH

THERE ARE MANY PROFESSIONALS (or pseudoprofessionals)
currently promoting everything from eating healthy foods to
avoiding toxins. We see them on television, hear them on the
radio, visit their colorful websites, and read their books. Some
make a lot of sense. Some make no sense at all. Some are sincere.
Others only want to make a buck.

A few stress balance, but most harp on their area of interest as
if nothing else matters. Then they drive home their message with
a polished and convincing sales pitch. Some give good information. Others present partial truths. All proclaim they have found
the answer. *The* answer. If only it were that simple.

How do we put all this information together in a way that
makes sense? How do average people who live average lives know
what to believe, whom to believe, or what the next step should
be? Do we wait for a governmental regulation or the family
physician to tell us what to do? Do we take personal responsibility? Do the answers really exist?

Take high-fructose corn syrup. We hear that it's killing us. Surely our government would not allow it on the market, and our local hospitals wouldn't be serving it to patients if this were true. When we take in this ingredient in our food, our bodies do not make leptin, which is a chemical that makes us feel full; therefore, we eat more than we should. Yet high-fructose corn syrup is listed among the ingredients of some of our favorite foods and neatly tucked inside many of the selections on the hospital menu.

We hear that argon is a chemical applied to fruits and vegetables to make them look great but it may do us a great deal of harm. Yet the fruits and vegetables we find in many grocery stores are coated with argon. What's going on?

Of course, I cannot address every bad food, dangerous toxin, dubious treatment, or deception out there, but I can give you a framework and approach to use as you face these apparent contradictions.

The first thing you should know is that by discovering what the body needs, you can uncover a lot about what the body doesn't need. For instance, there must be something about water that the body needs. We know this because, without a steady and sufficient supply of water, we would die. So we can safely conclude that food with low water content may not be what's best for us. True, our bodies can extract water from whatever food we eat, but here's an interesting fact. While most Americans are overweight, we are also severely dehydrated. This indicates that what most of us eat—and drink—doesn't contain the water we need. So if we're thirsty, we can just know that our bodies aren't asking us for a soft drink, a shot of whiskey, or a juicy steak. But what do many of us do when we're thirsty? We put the absolutely wrong things into our bodies.

The second thing to do is look in the mirror. To paraphrase a popular television psychologist, "How's that standard American diet working for you?" We've got to conclude that much of what we as a society are dumping into our bodies is wrong. Our diet is not helping us live healthy lives. As a matter of fact, the foods we eat are hurting us in more ways than I can count.

Third, truth does exist. But it is not necessarily where you think it is. While I agree with many of the professionals out there, I want to go one step further. Yes, I will talk about high-fructose corn syrup, preservatives, and the toxins in the world. But where did the ideas about healthy living come from in the first place? Who set the standard? Who created what I call "the ultimate prescription"?

Throughout this book, I want to tell you not only about why you have a problem but also about how you can find the ultimate prescription for it. The answers include a lot more than the foods you eat or the time you spend immobile in front of TV screens or computer monitors. It also includes the thoughts you think, who or what you worship, and how willing you are to love and be loved.

The answers, my friend, exist. They are the major part of the journey I traveled with David. But as with most major journeys, I needed to move slowly, one step at a time.

The Journey Begins

Once David was out of immediate danger, I had a chance to sit down with him and try to explain exactly what he'd been through.

Blockage of the arteries supplying the heart with blood is termed "coronary artery disease" or simply CAD. The problem develops because the coronary arteries become narrowed or completely blocked by plaque. When this occurs, blood, with its life-sustaining load of oxygen, can't reach the heart muscle. Without oxygen, the heart begins to "suffocate" and will eventually stop pumping.

What causes the arteries to be clogged? Your body carries fats called lipids in the blood. Lipids can gradually build up inside the blood vessels. These buildups can become hardened, or calcified. Then other factors become involved, making the blockages bigger and bigger. Blood has an increasingly difficult time passing through the arteries. That was the situation David was in when he was rushed to the hospital. He was experiencing an acute problem that needed immediate, acute care.

One thing to keep in mind is that plaque buildup can be occurring in any artery anywhere in the body, including the brain, the aorta, or the legs. Developing hand in hand with this buildup is inflammation or increased swelling within the arteries.

Sometimes a blockage, which is also called a "plaque mat," can become unstable. If this mat, which I sometimes think of as a pimple, pops, there can be big problems, even if there's only a 30 to 40 percent narrowing in the artery. The body sees this rupture as an injury and sends what it believes to be healing cells to the site.

If you cut your arm, many different types of cells are recruited to fight the damage. The same thing happens inside the artery when a plaque mat ruptures. The cells rushing to the rescue mean to do the body good, and usually, that's what they do. But at the mat rupture site, they do something less than helpful. They finish plugging up what space remains in the artery. The result? Blood flow is stopped, and the owner of the artery experiences a debilitating heart attack.

How many of us are going through life thinking everything is just fine when, unseen and unfelt, something is building inside us—something dangerous and life threatening?

I went on to explain to David that unfortunately, there are no diagnostic tests to predict which plaques will rupture. If we had such a test, we could predict heart attacks. When David's plaque "popped," the recruited damage-fighting cells formed a clot that resulted in a great restriction of blood flow in the artery. Severe pain from a heart muscle not receiving enough blood immediately followed.

The cornerstone in the acute treatment of CAD is first to restore blood flow to the heart as quickly as possible. Time lost is muscle lost. If the blocked artery is not opened quickly and the blood flow restored, a full heart attack will occur. Because of the lack of blood flow to the heart, the body's electrical system could be damaged and malfunction, resulting in a dangerously slow, fast, or uneven heart rhythm. When these rhythms occur, the heart may not be able to pump sufficient blood to the other organs of the body, and these organs also can begin to malfunction.

In addition to all this, the heart valves controlling the direction of blood flow depend on muscles that may be damaged during a heart attack. So now there's blood flowing—but in the wrong direction!

Most severe of all, during a heart attack, it is even possible that a dead heart muscle may break open or rupture. This situation is usually fatal.

By this time, David was shaking his head in utter amazement. He'd felt nothing until that attack. He didn't know it was coming. "So, Dr. Marcum," he said. "This plaque. Where did it come from?"

There are times in life when the truth bites like a lion. This was one of those times. "David," I said, "the stressors in your life, the cigarettes you smoked, the foods you ate, and the genetic bombs you triggered with your unhealthy lifestyle caused it."

Sources of Plaque

Remember when I mentioned lipids a few paragraphs back? Lipids are the fats that create plaque. What I didn't say was where they came from.

A lipid is an oily organic compound that is insoluble in water and, along with proteins and carbohydrates, is an essential structural component of every living cell. In other words, lipids are good. Our cells need them to be cells. These fats, or lipids, need to be ingested.

In our diet, there are two sources of lipids—animal products and plant products. Both deliver fats to the body. So the only way to supply our bodies with lipids is to eat them.

But here's the problem: animal products contain high levels of fat. As a matter of fact, some, like cheese, are almost entirely fat.

Plant foods, on the other hand, are very low in fat, providing just enough for cell development and maintenance. So when I toss out a statistic like "It has been estimated that 82 percent of heart attacks that occur before the age of sixty-five could be prevented," one of the main elements of that statistic is diet.

Think of all the lives that could be saved if people knew what I just said. But they don't know. Why? Because the meat industry is a multibillion-dollar conglomerate able to mount incredibly expensive advertising campaigns convincing us that meat is good for us, that milk is good for us, that pork is good for us.

When was the last time you watched a "carrots are good for you" commercial on television? When was the last time you heard, "Where's the spinach?" so often that it became a cultural catchphrase? When was the last time you read in a popular magazine an ad that headlined the words, "Got soy?"

Excess fat in the body, just like excess tension, excess guilt, excess stimulation of any kind, stresses the organs, including the heart. These stresses can be totally hidden, working unseen and unfelt deep inside us, causing our systems to malfunction and, as in David's case, almost shut down completely.

The concept of food as a stressor may be a new idea for many people. It was to David. All those hamburgers, all those deep-fried fries, all those juicy steaks and barbecued ribs, all those bowls of ice cream and frosty glasses of milk placed unseen and unfelt stresses on his body as they provided the building blocks for a steady buildup of plaque. Then came the tipping point, with its unbearable pain and the race to the hospital. Now David had his stent. The blood was flowing again. But the problem wasn't fixed. What we had been able to do was simply give David another chance to fix it himself.

David was very, very fortunate. But his journey was far from over.

IF YOU THINK YOU'RE HAVING A HEART ATTACK . . .

If you think you are having a heart attack, here's what you need to do. Sit down, call 911, and leave the phone off the hook so your call can be traced if you get too weak to talk or you pass out. If possible, take an aspirin, and try your best to relax. *Do not* drive yourself to the emergency room. If a friend or neighbor, instead of the paramedics, takes you to the hospital, as soon as you arrive, let everyone know that you think you are having a heart attack. This is no time to sit down in the waiting room and patiently wait your turn. If you are having feelings you can't explain, the sooner you seek help the better.

3

ASKING WHY

THE NUMBERS are staggering. Researchers at the National Coalition on Health Care believe that by 2017, health care may account for $4.3 trillion in annual spending—a fifth of every dollar needed to keep our economy running.

Right now, the direct and indirect cost of smoking rings in at $193 billion per year according to the Centers for Disease Control and Prevention. Diabetes cost this country $116 billion in 2007, and heart disease lifted $305 billion from the nation's coffers in 2009 for acute services, medications, and lost productivity. Obesity? Our girth isn't the only thing that's being supersized. Treating this condition and the cascade of diseases for which it opens doors is draining $147 billion annually from our collective savings accounts.

But as staggering as the above statistics are, the issue, for me, is not really money. It's the tears I see in so many eyes, the distorted sounds that echo in my stethoscope, the troubling images that emerge from MRIs, CAT scans, and X-ray machines that create the greatest concern in my mind. People are suffering, and in so many cases, that suffering is self-imposed, not from living their lives in defiance of sound health laws, but from living in ignorance of them. David was just such a case.

During my follow-up visits with him, I began to realize something interesting. When it came to knowing how to properly care for the human body, my search for truth was, in many ways, paralleling his search.

Medical school had done a terrific job of preparing me for the most effective ways to treat acute illnesses. I had become extremely adept at keeping people alive using the amazing tools of the cardiology profession. I could rapidly diagnose a heart problem and apply what was needed to keep my patient's family from having to cash in his or her life insurance policy. But as I began to see my patients returning to me with the very same conditions time and time again, I realized my training had not gone far enough. I'd become a doctor to make people well, not just to keep them from dying.

Many years ago, when I was a medical resident, I helped take care of a man with a malignancy. The medical team in charge of his care thought that a bone marrow transplant was the way to go. So we began blasting him with powerful chemotherapy to kill the malignant cells. As is usually the case with such procedures, this treatment also killed off many of his good cells. I remember watching his white and red blood cell count drop as his bone marrow succumbed to the powerful chemotherapy. We had to give him transfusions and then load him up with various antibiotics at the faintest sign of infection.

The man suffered greatly under the treatment. The medications made him sick. He was nauseated most of the time. But our patient was courageous even though he was isolated in a sterile room, could see his family for only limited periods, and was constantly bombarded with the best that modern medicine had to offer.

Soon it was time for the bone marrow transplant. Hopes ran high that the malignancy was gone. Yes, he was gaining strength, but the strain on his systems had left him looking much older than his real age. While I was amazed at the science and technology surrounding the case, deep down I felt something was missing. Our hopes, the patient's hopes, the patient's family's hopes, were all tied into what modern medicine could do—and I was part of that.

Not long after the marrow transplant, my patient became desperately ill. A sudden infection gripped his body in a terrible embrace, and despite the use of ventilators, dialysis, and intravenous medications and nutrition, he died.

As he was nearing the end, I was in his room caring for him. I remember him looking at me with unspoken questions in his eyes, but he passed away before I could provide any answers. This bothered me a great deal. Everything I knew—everything that modern medicine had to offer—was not enough to save him. That's when I turned to God with that same look in my eyes. There had to be more—more information, more insights, more truth than what I'd been taught at medical school. Right then and there I prayed for God to open my eyes, help me find truth, and give me the courage to speak out when others were silent.

And so began a slow journey that continues to this day. I started looking beyond my medical textbooks for answers. Ultimately, I began searching for healing truth where most people search for spiritual truth—in the pages of God's Holy Word. What I found was astonishing.

Why?

The first thing I did in my search for understanding of disease was to begin asking the all-important and often overlooked question, Why? Why is this heart sick? Why is this person short of breath? Why is my patient suffering such debilitating pain? Why does a disease that just a few years ago attacked only the elderly now challenge this young person? Why does the human body react this way or that way? Why are cardiovascular diseases, diabetes, obesity, and cancer rates soaring to such incredible heights? We were not created to be sick. Experiencing a heart attack wasn't part of the original plan God had in mind for His created beings.

I wanted something concrete—something unchanging on which to base my mode of operation as a physician.

As I searched, I found it becoming painfully obvious that we are being influenced into thinking that understanding *why* is not important. Voices keep telling us that truth doesn't matter, that we should simply let someone else tell us how or what to think. We are being told to let television, radio, the Internet think for us. If a doctor or preacher says it, it *must* be true. In other words, we don't need to understand why things happen. We just need to accept them as inevitable facts of life and go on as best we can.

But those same voices keep tripping over themselves. "This medicine is great," I hear them proclaim. Then, just as my patients are almost adjusted to that particular brand's side effects, I read about it being pulled off the market—something about people dying.

"A low-fat diet is good," I hear. Then, "No, actually high carb is the way to go!"

"Caffeine is good."

"Caffeine is bad."

In our heavily marketed world, how does one know whom or what to believe? Allow me to be brutally honest: too many people are making money at the expense of others. Our good health is not the driving force behind many products today. Our ignorance is. Unscrupulous companies are depending on our being too uninformed or simply too busy to know the truth. In essence, we are being held captive by our own lack of interest in the question, Why?

One of the first Bible texts that caught my attention as I began studying that very question was this gem: "You will know the truth, and the truth will set you free" (John 8:32). That is what I wanted. I wanted to be free from hype and tradition. I wanted my interaction with patients to be based on healing advice, not profitable prescriptions. While I was certainly prepared to deal with any acute condition that came my way, I wanted to make sure that when my patients left my office, they would have real information that could be used to deal effectively with their conditions. I didn't want to see them coming back to me in a few months suffering from a new malady brought on by an old disease. I wanted them cured. Yes, I wanted their problem *fixed*.

Stress as a Cause of Disease

Emily is sixty-four years old. Her children are grown and married and living in different states. But her life is far from peaceful. Her eighty-six-year-old mother suffers from Alzheimer's disease, and Emily has been the woman's sole caregiver for the past five years. Daily she feeds her mother, bathes her, gives her medications, points out the date, and even explains to her, time and time again, that, yes, she is her daughter.

Over the past four years, Emily has given up most of her social life, and her marriage has suffered because she spends most of her time in the caregiver mode. Unfortunately, the family doesn't possess the resources to use a special care facility.

What Emily—and the thousands like her that must face this type of situation—doesn't know is that her stressful life could very well be changing the chemical environment within her body. This stress could cause any number of illnesses. That's right. The life Emily is living could make her very, very sick.

The dictionary defines *stress* as the physical, chemical, or emotional factor that causes bodily or mental tension and may be a factor in disease. Originally, we were designed by God to live stress free—no selfishness, no disease, no clueless bosses or unrepentant enemies, no wayward children or disenfranchised spouses, no having to explain to your own mother who you are. We were created to live in a perfect, love-filled world.

But as time advanced, we had greater and greater levels of stress placed on our bodies. Now we even have to carry the heavy genetic load of stress passed down to us from previous generations. Add to that factors such as polluted environments, toxic foods, and information overload and you can see how far we have drifted from that original stress-free plan.

The body's response to stress can involve more than fourteen hundred chemical reactions utilizing up to thirty different hormones and neurotransmitters (substances that transmit nerve impulses). And these are only the reactions we know about!

We have all heard of the stress hormone epinephrine, also called adrenaline. When we are under stress, the body releases this chemical, which places us in the so-called "fight-or-flight" mode. This isn't necessarily a bad thing. If you saw a rattlesnake in the road, ready to strike, adrenaline would kick in and you'd jump back. We've all heard stories of people having supernatural strength in stressful situations while the body is pumping out adrenaline at high levels.

Epinephrine is released by the adrenal glands, as is a sister hormone, norepinephrine. When these chemicals are released, nerves throughout the body—using something called the "sympathetic nervous system"—are activated. What occurs next is a miracle. Your heart rate increases as needed. Your heart pumps more blood, rushing increased levels of oxygen to the body. Your blood vessels constrict, diverting blood to your muscles and brain and away from your skin and digestive tract. Under these extreme and temporary conditions, your muscles can do more, lift more, and react faster. Your brain is quicker, too, reaching conclusions rapidly on how to address the problem. Your pupils dilate so you can see better—even in low-light situations. Sugars and fats are moved into your blood to supply added energy. Your blood clots faster if there's bleeding, and your brain becomes very focused.

But there's more. Cortisol is released, which stimulates the delivery of fuel for energy. Cortisol is usually secreted in a twenty-four-hour pattern, highest in the morning and lowest around midnight. But in times of stress, it's made available in high amounts *right now*.

As I said, this is all fine and good if there's a rattlesnake in your path. But we as a society seem to be having a lot more than poisonous snakes getting in our way. We have bumper-to-bumper traffic, psychotic coworkers, rude neighbors, demanding bosses, and disrespectful children. Our fight-or-flight mode is switched on almost constantly. That means that all the special functions I listed above are engaged constantly. That's just not right. More to the point, that's just not healthy.

When the body is under chronic stress from whatever the cause, cortisol levels, for instance, remain elevated. If these levels are high at night, sleep is disturbed, the body cannot rest, and more stress is added to the system. High levels of cortisol cause extra insulin production, and the body responds to this by *storing* fat instead of burning fat. This buildup of fat, called the endocannabinoid system, generates its own hormones and chemical environment, which puts more stress on the body by the stimulation of inflammation. Chronic inflammation, in turn, is a stressor leading to many dangerous conditions, including heart disease.

The point is that acute stress and its chemical reactions are needed responses from time to time. But chronic stress damages the system via a host of chemical reactions involving the entire body—the mind, the cardiovascular system, even metabolism. In short, our entire beings are impacted by the stress under which we all seem to be living these days. So there's little wonder that we're facing skyrocketing rates of obesity, diabetes, high blood pressure, heart attacks, irregular heart rhythms, insomnia, infections (stress chemistry weakens the immune system), depression, inflammation, and the list goes on and on and on. All can be traced to the chemistry of chronic stress.

The Sad Truth

The sad truth is that the world—including the health care industry—does not relieve a state of chronic stress. No one goes around saying this out loud, but think about it. Remove stress, and you remove the cause of most diseases. No chronic stress means no need for all those pills, potions, doctor visits, surgeries, therapy sessions, and endless research that addresses the results of being stressed out.

This thought formed a turning point in my career. Instead of chasing after symptoms, I decided the best way to really make people whole again was to chase down the cause of their sicknesses. If I knew why they were sick, I could do much more good than simply trying to make them comfortable in their sickness.

Did it ever cross my mind that if I taught my patients how not to get sick, they wouldn't need me anymore? Certainly. But I also knew that it's human nature to resist change—even if ultimately that change is good for you. There would always be people who refused to change, and I wanted to be there for them, too. But those willing to follow my lead could begin making real changes in their lives—changes that would reduce or eliminate their need for much of modern medicine.

So when David stepped into my office for our next follow-up visit, I was ready for him. Whether he liked it or not, I was going to find out what was stressing his system and then teach him how to eliminate all possible stressors. My goal was that, eventually, I would never have to see him again—as his doctor.

4

HIDDEN STRESSES

"David, do you take a shower every day?"

My patient stared at me for a moment. "Yes, Dr. Marcum," he said, squirming uneasily in his chair. "Is there a reason you asked that particular question?"

I laughed. "No, you're very clean."

"Are you saying that taking a daily shower is a good treatment for heart disease?"

"Well, not exactly," I said. "Although it would probably improve many people's social lives. I just wanted to know your response so I could ask you another question. How do you feel if you miss a shower for a day or two?"

David grinned shyly. "Smelly. Grungy."

I folded my patient's chart and tossed it on my desk. "The point I'm trying to make is, there are certain things we need to do daily in order to accomplish something important. For instance, you shower every day to stay clean and not offend anyone by body odor, right?"

"Right."

"And it's probably safe for me to say that you use water for your shower instead of, oh, soda pop or honey."

David nodded. "I try to stay away from cranberry juice and gasoline, too."

"Right," I chuckled. "You use water because water is the only thing that really cleans the human body. Add a touch of soap, perhaps a rubber ducky, and you're good to go. Squeaky clean. No odor. All because of water."

My patient eyed me suspiciously. "Something tells me there's a broader point to this conversation," he said.

I picked up his chart again and started leafing through it. "Can I be honest with you?" I asked.

"I wouldn't expect anything else from the man who saved my life. Fire away!"

I paused and studied my patient for a long moment. "David, you're taking better care of your outside than your inside. You always come into my office dressed in clean clothes, with your hair combed, teeth brushed, shoes shined. Yet you're ignoring what's inside. Outside you look great. Inside, you're a total mess."

David frowned. "What do you mean?"

"Well, let's stay with water. When was the last time you enjoyed a great big glass of pure, unadulterated water just because you wanted to? Is there a big water jug in your refrigerator at home waiting to quench your thirst? Do you carry a water bottle around with you just in case you get a little parched on the job?"

David shook his head. "Water is boring," he said. "Who drinks that?"

"Not very many people," I responded. "As a matter of fact, it's been estimated that up to 70 percent of us Americans are dehydrated. And in that condition, an amazing amount of stress is brought on your body. Your heart works harder because your blood is thicker. Your brain doesn't think as clearly as it could because your sluggish blood is not delivering an optimum amount of oxygen to it. Your kidneys are working overtime trying to filter out impurities from your blood without having enough water to help flush those impurities out of your system. Your intestines and colon are bogged down, filled with by-products of digestion without a proper solution of water and fiber to move the waste material along. I could go on and on, but my point is that all these problems are associated directly with the fact that you're not drinking enough water. This is something you must do daily to accomplish something important for your entire body."

"So, if I drink more water, my heart problem would go away?"

"It's certainly a step in the right direction, but there's more. A lot more."

It All Comes Down to Stress

As a doctor, I'm always challenged to find ways of getting my patients to see the bigger picture when it comes to their health. And the truth is, it all comes down to stress—stress on the organs, stress on the brain, stress on the blood supply, stress on the heart. Many times, my patients don't even realize that they're bringing almost unbearable stress upon their bodies.

Today it's common knowledge that smoking—and secondhand smoke—are huge sources of chronic stress on the human physiology. But many people still smoke. Inadequate rest produces enormous amounts of stress as well, yet we are sleeping about two hours less per night than our great-grandfathers did.

Then there's our environment. We are filling our homes with smells we were never designed to sample. Synthetic perfumes and "lightly scented" toiletries and laundry soaps are introducing into our bodies elements that—to be blunt—are poison.

We take perfectly good foods and process the nutrients right out of them, leaving a bland and colorless product that requires copious amounts of additives such as salt and sugar to make them even palatable. What we can't process, we ignore.

Being overweight places an incredible amount of stress on the human body. Here's an interesting point to ponder: as we gain weight, we don't gain structure. The very same bones that support a 160-pound man are called on to support him when he weighs 360 pounds. No, we were not designed to be fat. If we're overweight, we're doing something terribly wrong to our bodies. Yet obesity rates are hovering at dangerous levels.

Consider our delicate digestive systems. They accept food, extract the needed nutrients, make energy available to the muscles, and basically fuel our lives. But we keep dumping this vital fuel into our systems exactly when we don't need it—in the evening before we go to bed. Then we don't fuel ourselves exactly when we do need it most—in the morning before we head off to work or school or whatever other activities fill our days.

Even water, that all-important ingredient to keeping us healthy, has become the beverage almost no one orders at a restaurant. If a waiter happens to place a glass in front of us, we might allow our dehydrated bodies a few sips before turning our attention to our favorite soda pop or alcoholic drink—both of which actually remove what little water we have in our blood in order to neutralize their high acidity as they enter our bodies. That same water that cleans us so well on the outside is the perfect beverage to clean us on the inside, yet we ignore it and call it boring.

When it comes to our minds, we are not being all that diligent there either. A bad work environment, memories we can't seem to escape, unrelenting anger, soul-scarring grief, unresolved guilt, and endless loneliness all work in concert to add extreme stress to our whole being. Toss in a couple of divorces, sour relationships, and a life dependent on a bank's credit line and, well, look around at the crowded doctors' offices and pharmacies. You get the picture. These hidden stresses are sucking the health right out of our minds and bodies, filling them instead with the valueless junk of fast food, fast times, and fast-working diseases. Our illnesses aren't killing us. *We're* killing us. Disease is often just a symptom of a life being lived out of step with the reality of how we were designed to live.

"There you go again," David said as I returned to my seat behind my desk. "Designed to live. *Designed to live.* How can we know how we were designed to live? We weren't made in a factory somewhere. We didn't come with an owner's manual."

"That's where you're wrong, David," I said, as gently as I could. "I know exactly where we came from, and yes, we do have an owner's manual. But people don't talk much, if at all, about that. No one seems to be writing about it or preaching about it or singing songs about it. It has to be the best-kept secret in the world."

David looked at me skeptically. "Okay, Doc," he said. "Write me a prescription for it, and I'll pick it up on my way home. It is covered by my medical plan, right?"

I smiled. "Tell you what," I said as I walked my patient to the door. "During our next visit, I'll give you one free. No charge."

My patient blinked. "A doctor giving out free meds? This I gotta see."

As I watched David walk down the hall, I thought about our conversation. Throughout time, physicians have wanted to blame one agent or another as the possible cause of illness and cardiovascular disease. A meat-rich diet, cigarettes, high blood pressure, and more recently, high cholesterol levels have been implicated in heart disease. Physicians are now looking at inflammation as the smoking gun. I wish it were that simple.

I wish I could say to someone, "Your genetics say you'll get heart disease, so you may as well start taking statins now. As a matter of fact, let's just put statins in our water supply so everyone is safe." Don't laugh. It's been discussed.

Besides making a few pharmaceutical companies very, very happy—and even richer than they are now—such a radical approach to heart disease would do nothing to stem the tide. Heart disease is still the number one killer in America and is a growing problem worldwide, in spite of the fact that we've been doling out powerful medicines designed to combat it for years. The bottom line is that *stress* causes heart disease. The chronic stressors we allow into our lives build up until our bodies are overwhelmed with adverse chemistry. Then a symptom develops. Sometimes, tragically, the first symptom is a full-blown heart attack. That was the case with David.

While a minority of patients suffer from purely genetic problems such as congenital abnormalities, including bad heart valves, certain abnormal heart rhythms, and even weak hearts, most cardiovascular disease is acquired. When we put chronic stress on the system, damage occurs, and then we look to modern medicine to bring us back from the brink. Sometimes it can; often it can't.

In today's world, it's not only the patient's heart that's broken. It's our health system as well.

Perpetuating Illness

If I were trying to perpetuate illness in the world, I would sneak just enough truth into the popular media and modern medical practices to make it believable, add some good marketing techniques to convince people that modern medicine can cure their ills, and then make my fortune treating symptoms with expensive pills and procedures. Next I'd throw in some special medicines that numbed the senses just enough to make people think their problem was solved. I'd try to figure out ways to get people to turn to other people—or even the government—for truth. I'd use the media to control minds and discourage patients from thinking or asking questions. I'd encourage society to be too busy—even doing good things—to think at all.

Then I'd convince religious denominations to become politically active machines, bent on preserving certain belief systems by urging members to become judgmental, legalistic, and overly indoctrinated. When it came to health care, I'd have impressive and sophisticated high-tech devices and treatments delivered by intelligent people.

In the natural world, I would encourage folks to look to certain foods, or parts of foods, that provide medicinal benefits (e.g., nutraceuticals), specific herbs, or some New Age theory as a cure for *all* their problems, and I'd use the power of the Internet to present and support my claims.

Finally, I'd slowly poison people with palate-pleasing foods— foods that destroy the environment during their production. I'd encourage people to exhaust themselves, making the fast-paced, grab-it-while-you-can, everything-all-the-time lifestyle their ultimate goal. Then I'd sprinkle in a few wars, natural disasters, new taxes, and be on my way. Last, I would never want people to ask why.

The horror of it all is that what I've just described is exactly what is happening in this world. It's precisely the mode of operation of some unseen, unrecognized power that is moving among us like a dark shadow. I had promised David a free prescription for his heart disease. I had to deliver on my promise. After months of searching for answers, I felt I had something to offer. He'd asked for an owner's manual for his body. And I was bound and determined to give him one.

5

DEADLY MISCONCEPTIONS

WE'VE GOT A PROBLEM in this country—a serious, life-threatening problem. And it's coming from the very industry on which we depend during our times of illness.

I'm a medical doctor—a board-certified cardiologist to be exact. I use powerful medications to treat acute cases of cardiovascular disease every day. Without the proper administration of these pharmaceuticals, many of my patients could die.

The problem I'm talking about stems from the mistaken belief that these medications contain healing powers. They don't. At best, they have the ability to sidetrack a problem, to work around it in order to keep a person alive long enough so that actual healing can take place. And when administered properly, these medications can do some pretty amazing things.

But when you move out of the emergency room, out of the acute-care ward, drugs become anything but your best friend. Let me ask you a few questions. How often do you leave a doctor's office with a new prescription tucked neatly into your purse or wallet? How often do you stand in line at the drugstore, waiting for that magical paper sack that contains what your physician says will deal effectively with your latest ailment? How much did you—and your health insurance plan—pay for what's in that sack?

For all the money you just spent, for all the years of training your doctor underwent, for all the safeguards built into the pharmaceutical system by our very own Food and Drug Administration (FDA), you'd think that what you were about to drop down your throat or inject into your skin would be safe. Think again.

In the *Morbidity and Mortality Weekly Report* released in 2007 by the Centers for Disease Control and Prevention (CDC) (available at www.cdc.gov/mmwr), researchers reported that "deaths from prescription drugs rose from 4.4 per 100,000 people in 1999 to 7.1 per 100,000 in 2004. This increase represents a jump from 11,000 people to almost 20,000 in the span of five years. Among the 20,000 that died, more than 8,500— double the number from 1999—were from 'other and unspecified drugs.' Psychotherapeutic drugs, like antidepressants and sedatives, nearly doubled from 671 deaths to 1,300."

In a landmark study titled "Death by Medicine," released in 2003, authors Gary Null, PhD; Carolyn Dean, MD; Martin Feldman, MD; Debora Rasio, MD; and Dorothy Smith, PhD, added fuel to the fire. "A definitive review and close reading of medical peer-review journals and government health statistics shows that American medicine frequently causes more harm than good. . . . The number of people having in-hospital, adverse drug reactions to prescribed medicine is 2.2 million. Dr. Richard Besser, of the CDC, in 1995 said the number of unnecessary antibiotics prescribed annually for viral infections was 20 million. Dr. Besser, in 2003, now refers to tens of millions of unnecessary antibiotics. The number of unnecessary medical and surgical procedures

performed annually is 7.5 million. The number of people exposed
to unnecessary hospitalization annually is 8.9 million. The total
number of iatrogenic [inadvertent physician-induced] deaths is
783,936. It is evident that the American medical system is the
leading cause of death and injury in the United States. The 2001
heart disease annual death rate is 699,697; the annual cancer
death rate, 553,251." The abstract of this study is available online
(http://www.healthe-livingnews.com/articles).

According to these numbers, you're more likely to die from
the treatment than from the disease itself. Yet we continue to
spend billions of dollars each year seeking cures by prescription.
Something is terribly wrong.

So, who's going to fix the problem? I doubt it will be our
governmental agencies. There are far too many lobbyists and
companies willing to donate enormous amounts of money to
those in power. The media? It's not likely. There are too many
advertising dollars to be made. Physicians? Who wants the
hassle—and the criticism? Attorneys? Nope. Medical lawsuits
earn them millions each year.

That leaves you and me—ordinary citizens. But first, we have
to identify the misconceptions about medications, know where
they came from, and how best to overturn their influence in our
lives. Until we do, we remain victims of our own ignorance.

Again, let me say clearly that some medications are needed.
But all medications produce stress on the human body, and we
must take care to weigh the risks versus the benefits of their use.
For instance, doctors are writing endless prescriptions for antibiotics while viruses are becoming more and more drug resistant.
Why are they becoming drug resistant? Because of all the antibiotics we're taking.

We're overprescribing acid-blocking medications. But stomach acid is a great defense against unwanted bacterial "bugs."

And patients on these medications can double their chances of developing pneumonia and diarrhea. These commonly prescribed medications—as well as their over-the-counter cousins—also decrease calcium absorption, thus tripling the risk of hip fractures. Yet many of these same medications boast "calcium added" in their promotions. They've included the very thing that their presence interrupts.

What about sleeping pills? Those who take them regularly experience a fivefold increase in cognitive defects, along with more daytime fatigue. Those pills knock you out, but they don't provide the needed rest.

This list could go on to include memory-enhancing pills, certain medications for dementia, and some diabetes prescriptions, but I think you get the picture. Drugs are not always what they seem to be.

So what do we do? What do I as a physician do? That's the question I asked myself years ago as I began to realize that what I was doing for people wasn't helping them in the long run. I was keeping my patients alive long enough for their disease or condition to regroup and attack again. This was a great business plan, but I knew something "big" was missing, and I was determined to find out what.

An Answer

I was born and raised in a Christian home. I attended church, sang hymns, read my Bible, and prayed. But for some reason, I never saw a connection between those activities and health. More to the point, I never connected those activities to the *building and maintaining* of health. Christianity was something I *did*, something I *believed*, not something I used to stay healthy.

But all that changed when I began to see a convergence taking place, a coming together of two elements—biblical theology and science. As scientists gained the tools necessary to peer further and further into what makes life possible, I found that what I read in my faithful Bible began to make more sense, as if modern researchers were seeking proof to verify what the Bible teaches. Study after study seemed to underline certain passages, bringing to light the Bible's ancient truths. This merging of science and the Bible changed the way I regarded Scripture and launched me on a search for healing that continues to this day. I realized that for the first time in history, science wasn't refuting the Bible's truth—it was proving it!

Health and good chemistry weren't just about eating the right foods and getting sufficient exercise. They were not just about pills versus plants or organic versus conventional. There are many treatments out there for every condition known to humans, but something much more important needed to be emphasized.

In my own search for truth, I came to realize that health is a by-product, an end result, of a love relationship with God. It begins with His loving us, and it ends with us loving Him. Everything else—every choice we make, every bad habit we overcome, every thought we think—must be a direct result of that growing connection we enjoy with the One who created us.

Follow me closely for a moment. The further we move away from that connection, the sicker we become, and the more stress we have on our systems. Originally, we were designed to worship God and become like what we worship. For optimal health and well-being, it's essential that we know the Great Physician. This is the way we were made to operate. When we worship anything else—money, power, technology, modern medicine, food, sports, movie stars, religious institutions, television, the Internet (the list goes on and on)—we move away from the original plan, and stress chemistry appears. That type of worship was not in the original design.

The further away we move from that connection, the sicker

we become. I knew that if I was going to help David find real, lasting healing, I'd have to connect him with the God he'd rejected and with the kind of life God had created him to live. As the day of David's next appointment approached, I turned to God as never before. Our next meeting would be critical to David's long-term healing process.

A Second Chance

It was obvious to me that David was improving. He was following some simple suggestions I had made concerning diet and exercise, and his chemistry was changing right before my eyes. He'd lost a little weight, his cholesterol was edging downward, and his heartbeat sounded much stronger and more regular. Blood pressure was heading back into the normal range, and the pungent smell of cigarette smoke was barely noticeable on him now. I made a few notations on his chart and then studied him thoughtfully.

"So," he said with a smile, "how'm I doin'?"

"You're doing well," I said. "But I want to remind you that—"

"I know. I'm not fixed. I'm just patched. I've got a lot more work to do."

I smiled. "You've been listening to me. I'm flattered!"

David grinned. "Hey, that little episode in here a month ago was kind of a wake-up call. I figure I've been given a second chance."

"I agree," I said, sitting down beside him. "And that's why I've got something for you. You can call it your 'second-chance kit.'"

"Oh, yeah," David said, beaming. "My free meds! I was hoping you hadn't forgotten."

I reached into a drawer in a nearby cabinet and withdrew

a small, rectangular package. "Here you go. Take two of these and call me in the morning."

Like a child at Christmas, David ripped open the packaging, then paused. "A Bible?" he exclaimed. "You're giving me a Bible?" He seemed disappointed.

"Good medicine," I said.

"Doc, I don't mean to sound ungrateful, but I'm not what you'd call a Christian. Bibles are for Christians, right?"

"Really?" I said. "The Bible is good for everybody. Christians have simply figured that out already."

My patient thought for a moment. "I . . . uh . . ."

"Listen, David," I said, leaning forward in my chair. "God didn't say what He said in this book because we love Him. He said what He said because He loves us. And because He loves us, He created laws that make life possible—and that includes, for example, the various laws of physics. If you jump off a building, you're going to fall. That's the law of gravity in full operation, whether or not you believe in it or in the God who created it.

"Well, that same God who created the law of gravity created a rather precise collection of laws that pertain directly to our health. Break a science law, and something bad usually happens. Break a health law, and you get sick. You stress your body. Your chemistry gets messed up. It's as simple as that."

"But how do I know the words in that Book are really true? How do I know those writings are not just an elaborate way the world has developed to cope with the inevitable—death?" David questioned.

"That is a great and relevant question," I responded. I explained to him that God spoke His message to us through mere humans, about forty writers, from about the time of Moses to around one hundred years after the birth of Christ. These people were His spokespersons.

Again David asked, "How do I know without doubt the words they spoke were from the God of the universe?"

"Well," I explained, "you could look at all the fulfilled prophecies, events predicted hundreds of years ahead of time. History shows all these events came to pass—from the rise of kingdoms like the Greek and Roman Empires predicted in the book of Daniel to the birth of Christ, foretold in great detail in the book of Isaiah. History has proved the Bible to be true—from the Dead Sea Scrolls, which contain fragments of many of the Bible books, to archaeological finds still being unearthed today. Science validates the Bible.

"David, I had similar questions at one time. The book *More Than a Carpenter*, by Josh McDowell, helped me when I needed proof that the Bible was true. You could read that little book."

I then added that what helped me most was something a wise person said to me during my searching moments: "'Don't let other people think for you. You can read all the material out there. You can talk to the most-educated people from both camps. But what I suggest is this: Give God a chance to prove that the Bible is true. Get a Bible and begin to read. Ask God to show you whether this Book really contains God's words or is just fiction. If you have an open mind and are sincere in your search, you will receive an answer.'

"This is the path I took, David," I continued. "As I began to communicate with God, He began to communicate with me and show me truth. The first truth was that I could depend on Him. When I did this, I could see Him leading in the events of my life. He was showing me not only that the Bible is true but that He loved me and wanted to be a part of my life.

"In a world where it's tough to know who or what to believe, I found the answer. I soon discovered the Bible also gives guidelines on the prevention and treatment of disease. When applied, these principles change the body's chemistry much like a pill or procedure but without the side effects and address the cause of the problem. In today's world this type of thinking is generally missing.

"Conversely, when we violate these biblical principles, we damage the body's fabric. I want my children, Kelli and Jake, to be healthy and make good decisions, because I love them and want them to be happy. God gives us suggestions in the Bible for the same reason. He loves us and wants us to be happy. The Creator is the real Master Physician, the One I want to listen to first."

David stiffened. "So you're saying that I had a heart attack because I was breaking some god's law? Well, excuse me. I thought you told me that I had my heart attack because I was smoking, eating too much fatty food, and not getting enough exercise. Where is it written, 'Thou shalt not smoke, eat junk food, or sit on your butt all day'?"

"I'm glad you asked that question, David," I said as I lifted the Bible from my patient's hand and turned to the very first pages. "If it's okay with you, I'd like to read you a story. And when we're finished, you can tell me why you had a heart attack."

David looked at me skeptically and then glanced down at the Bible as I began to read.

6

IN THE BEGINNING

WHEN I BEGAN to write this book, the Holy Spirit impressed me to write in a way that patterned Christ's ministry. Christ first met the physical needs of the people, restoring their sight, helping the lame to walk, or curing leprosy. He did not judge. He did not have a condescending attitude. He served.

After He met their acute needs, He then began to teach them truth using parables. Along the way, He revealed the mistaken beliefs of the time. He introduced them to love and the path to healing. His approach was available and understandable to everyone.

In the first part of this book, I've tried to introduce you to the problem. Remember, if you don't understand the problem, it's difficult to find the solution. David had a serious physical need when he had a heart attack. But after I had met that need, I began to teach him.

The problem, as we've discovered, is stress—stress on our genetics, stress from the foods we eat, stress in our thoughts, basically anything we do that goes against the way we were designed. This stress activates chemical changes that are damaging to the body and lead to symptoms of disease and the need for acute care. Stress has been in the world since almost the beginning, but it seems to be escalating in the times in which you and I live.

Now that we have a framework in regards to the problem, it is time to move on to talking about the solution.

First, I want to get something out in the open. I suspect that you know what's coming next, but I want to say it anyway. I believe in a God who created the world and also created the laws that govern it. I believe in a God who has the power to heal and has infused that power deep in our own bodies. Finally, I believe that God wants us all to be aware of and to utilize the gifts He has provided so that we can begin to overcome sickness of the mind, the body, and the spirit.

This may sound strange coming from a man of science, but it's true. While many in my profession focus entirely on the technological achievements, the amazing intellect of those who create that technology, and—for want of a better word—seem to *worship* the science behind medicine and healing, I feel they're missing something important.

If I'm having a heart attack, I want a skilled physician to implant a stent to open the blocked passage, and when I wake up from surgery, I'm going to be overjoyed that such science and technology are available. Even though medications and medication errors are leading causes of death, if I have a bacterial infection, I want an antibiotic. As I've said before, there's definitely a place for modern medicine. There always has been, and there always will be.

But I have also come to realize that disease does not just jump into the human body. In more cases than not, humans contribute to its being there. We're beginning to better understand the chemistry that drives both health and disease, and as that understanding increases, many of us in the scientific community are beginning to appreciate the logic behind what God did in creation. As a matter of fact, I have come to the place in my own life where "Creator logic" trumps human understanding every time. Even if I don't fathom why God did something, I know there must have been a reason, and I find great joy and satisfaction in searching for that reason.

When it comes to how we're supposed to interact with God, He doesn't ask for blind faith. To paraphrase the words of a popular gospel song some years ago, God never says, "I said it, and you believe it, and that should be good enough for you."

Our God is a logical, highly scientific Being. He doesn't work in the shadows or keep His cards close to His chest. In one of the most thrilling texts in the Bible, the One who made us invites, "'Come now, let's settle this,' says the Lord" (Isaiah 1:18). "I have nothing to hide," He seems to be saying. "I'll tell you everything you want to know."

Then we read this incredible statement. "I will guide you along the best pathway for your life. I will advise you and watch over you. Do not be like a senseless horse or mule that needs a bit and bridle to keep it under control" (Psalm 32:8-9). How many of us are being controlled by powers other than our own understanding? How many of us are bridled to the media, to the Internet, to some health fad that will soon be shown to be flawed, or even dangerous?

I want you to consider trusting God in a way you've never trusted Him before. I want you to begin worshiping the God who created science instead of worshiping at the altar of human interpretation of that science.

Hands-on God

As I mentioned earlier, many years ago I read a book by Josh McDowell titled *More Than a Carpenter*. It provides fascinating examples of events predicted in the Bible that were fulfilled over the centuries. The book presents case after case in which archaeology has proved the Bible's accuracy. This reinforced my belief in the God who not only created me but also had remained involved in the history leading up to my birth. This God is totally "hands on." He was—and is—always ready to reason with anyone willing to listen to Him.

Would that be you? Are you ready to listen?

Something else I discovered about God is that He can't lie. It's not just that He doesn't. He can't. He can't even tell a "white" lie because He's all about truth, and lying would violate His character. When He says something, it happens. Period.

As I was moving down this path during my college years at the University of Texas, I began recognizing that scientific and prophetic evidence were coming together to prove that the Bible is true. And in the process of gathering evidence, I found that I was also developing a relationship with God. Suddenly, God wasn't some distant power simply observing my progress through life. He became real to me—a force, a presence to whom I could turn when the questions got too big to bear.

This experience is what I want for my children. It's what I want for my patients. And it's what I want for you.

The Secret Is the Search

The story is told of a physics professor whose specialty was energy and matter. Year after year, in his classroom at the university, he opened up to his students the great mysteries of the universe, teaching them how matter could be turned into energy, how energy could make matter, and how speed and time were interrelated. He proposed a theory to explain how God could be at all places at all times based on the manipulation of speed and time. Even though his class was challenging, there was a waiting list of students hoping for a place at the professor's feet.

Open-minded students tended to do well. Status-quo seekers—those who simply wanted to memorize a bunch of words or concepts—usually had problems in the class and struggled for a passing grade. Not surprisingly, the administration was constantly giving the professor grief about his methods, but the results reflected in the lives of many who took his class, and the deep love they felt for the man served to produce strong arguments that he was truly on to something valuable.

Near the end of one semester, the professor informed his students that there would be a final physics test the following week. When the day arrived, those in the class sat expectantly, waiting to see what their instructor had in store for them. "Your final test for this class is a simple one," he announced. "I'm going to divide you up into teams and give you the chance to assemble this small automobile." He pulled the covering off a diminutive foreign car at the front of the class. "It's mostly assembled already and there's fuel in the tank. All you have to do is complete the assembly, start it, and drive it ten feet."

Then the professor held up a block of paraffin and seven blank keys. "Oh, and you'll have to create the key that starts the ignition. Good luck."

Each team was handed a test booklet with these additional guidelines: (1) Read these instructions first. (2) Remember the big picture in figuring out how to make this car run successfully. (3) Start by inflating the tires. (4) Move onto the fuel and other systems.

The students gathered in their teams and went over their challenge: blank keys, a block of paraffin, nearly assembled car, no questions to answer, no complex mathematical formulas to work, no calculus to use, no aerodynamics to ponder. Piece of cake!

The professor informed his students that they'd all make an A if they could get the car to start and drive it ten feet.

The students attacked the problem with enthusiasm. Some immediately hooked up the fuel system. Some tried to make keys by etching grooves in the blanks that had been provided. Still others checked the electrical system, making sure power was getting from the battery to the starter coil. One team even had the forethought to test the provided fuel, making sure it was the type that the engine needed.

At the end of the first hour, the car still sat there, engine quiet, and unmoving.

One student carefully watched the actions of the others, trying to fathom what the professor was attempting to teach with this unconventional test. He glanced over at the professor who sat at his big desk, watching the class thoughtfully. What was everyone missing? What were the students not doing right?

That's when his eyes fell on the instruction booklets laying scattered about the room. No one was reading them. No one was following the carefully printed guidelines.

The student picked up his copy and started to reread the professor's words. *(1) Read these instructions first.* Many had done that, but after reading, they'd simply headed off on their own paths, hoping that their own knowledge would solve the problems. *(2) Remember the big picture in figuring out how to make this car run successfully.* The student suddenly realized that the "big picture" included not only the car but also the instruction booklet. *(3) Start by inflating the tires.* A quick glance at the automobile's tires revealed that no one had done this. *Why inflate the tires of a car that can't run?*

The student walked over to the test car and began pumping

air into rubber. As the fourth tire swelled to full inflation, he noticed that something had been drawn on the sidewall— a finely detailed outline of . . . a key.

Wordlessly the student carefully copied that outline onto the paraffin wax, created an indentation in the wax based on the outline, strolled over to a heat source, melted several of the blank keys in a pan, and then poured the molten liquid into the paraffin outline. When the newly cast key had cooled, he lifted it out, brushed away the imperfections, got into the car, started the engine, and drove across the room.

In our world, our minds are being influenced, and often not for the better. We think we know the answers, but we don't. God does, and He's provided those answers in a very obvious place— His Holy Word. He hasn't hidden them. He hasn't locked them away from our searching eyes. But He does require something of us. If we want to discover how to "start" our journey back to optimum health and "drive" our lives to a satisfying end, we need to read—and follow—the simple guidelines He has provided.

In other words, you don't begin your journey back to health at your doctor's office. You don't search the Internet for answers to your most troubling questions. All this can come later. But first, you simply go to your bookshelf and retrieve the most sold but least read book this world has ever known. You sit down in a quiet place, open its pages, and begin to read. Because it's there that you'll discover the key to the change you've been longing to bring into your life.

As we continue to search for the solution, let's begin the journey together in the very first chapter of the first book of the Bible.

A Vision of Things to Come

On the sixth day of Creation week, God had spoken to Adam and Eve and said, "Be fruitful and multiply. Fill the earth and govern it. Reign over the fish in the sea, the birds in the sky, and all the animals that scurry along the ground" (Genesis 1:28). In other words, He's inviting the couple to care for His new creation, to nurture the land and love the animals—an assignment they apparently accept with great joy.

Then God says, "'Look! I have given you every seed-bearing plant throughout the earth and all the fruit trees for your food. And I have given every green plant as food for all the wild animals, the birds in the sky, and the small animals that scurry along the ground—everything that has life.' And that is what happened. Then God looked over all he had made, and he saw that it was very good!" (vv. 29-31).

Day seven had now arrived. I wish I could have been there in the very beginning. Try to imagine the scene with me. We see earth's first couple, fresh from the mind and hand of God, surrounded by a Garden teeming with life. I can picture the Creator joining the happy pair by a bubbling brook as they admired the flowers and animals on that seventh day of Creation. Surrounded by all that breathtaking beauty, God revealed something important to us all. It was now time to rest. "On the seventh day God had finished his work of creation, so he rested from all his work. And God blessed the seventh day and declared it holy, because it was the day when he rested from all his work" (Genesis 2:2-3). Everything Adam and Eve needed to live happy, healthy lives was right there in the Garden with them. More to the point, God's "Health Plan"—a plan constructed from pure love that would hold in perfect harmony this world and everything in it—was now in full effect, waiting to be enjoyed by every living thing. Nothing else was needed. In today's world, this is hard to imagine.

Here's what so many of us fail to realize today. That loving Health Plan is *still* in effect—*still* operating—and it is *still* the most powerful, concise, and effective way to build and maintain optimum health. That plan can still bring health and harmony to anyone's body, mind, and spirit.

By taking a careful look at the world as Adam and Eve saw it and as God created it, we can gain incredible insights into how we're supposed to live and into how we can survive in our fast-paced, anything-goes, if-it-feels-good-do-it world today. The laws that God set in place during those seven days of Creation are waiting to bring healing to our bodies, minds, and spirits today, no matter how much we've abused those principles in the past.

I've seen those laws of love at work in my patients—bringing healing when all else seemed to fail, changing their body's chemistry, relieving stress placed on their systems. Time and time again, the scientific community has proved that God's way is the best way—that His health laws are more powerful in dealing with and helping prevent chronic illnesses than any pharmaceuticals, medical devices, or high-tech procedures.

Most exciting of all, following God's health laws is inexpensive and universally applicable.

Would you like to know what those laws are? Would you like to discover what God had in mind for your body, your mind, and your relationship with your Creator? Let's spend some time digging into the story of Creation to discover those vital laws and to learn how to apply them to our lives today.

7

DAY 1—FROM DARKNESS TO LIGHT

IN THE BEGINNING GOD CREATED THE HEAVENS AND
THE EARTH. THE EARTH WAS FORMLESS AND EMPTY, AND
DARKNESS COVERED THE DEEP WATERS. AND THE SPIRIT OF
GOD WAS HOVERING OVER THE SURFACE OF THE WATERS.
THEN GOD SAID, "LET THERE BE LIGHT," AND THERE
WAS LIGHT. AND GOD SAW THAT THE LIGHT WAS GOOD.
THEN HE SEPARATED THE LIGHT FROM THE DARKNESS.
GOD CALLED THE LIGHT "DAY" AND THE DARKNESS "NIGHT."
AND EVENING PASSED AND MORNING CAME,
MARKING THE FIRST DAY.

—GENESIS 1:1-5

IT WAS NOW TIME to introduce David to the original plan for
health: the "owner's manual" I had given him. This plan is
perfect and was given to the world at Creation. It was designed
with you and me in mind. Unfortunately, a host of misconceptions that continue to this very day has sidetracked us. As we
have moved away from this plan, stress has entered our bodies at
every level. I needed to get David to understand the importance
of the original design.

When the Creator began His work, He didn't have a lot of
material at his disposal. Genesis 1:2 reveals that "the earth was

formless and empty, and darkness covered the deep waters." Not exactly a choice vacation spot. But there's more. There wasn't any light. I'm not talking about the absence of a sun or moon. I'm saying that light couldn't even exist there.

How is that possible? Well, have you ever heard of a black hole? Scientists are discovering more and more of these mysterious regions sprinkled throughout the known universe. Black holes are so dense, so packed with incredible power, so heavy with gravity, that light can't even exist in them. Perhaps the material that would soon become our world was floating around in the middle of a black hole when God began His transformations.

No one knows for sure how the Creator created, but the first thing He did was make light *possible* in the darkness. He spoke, and suddenly, there was light (see Genesis 1:3). The utter darkness that had gripped our world was gone with a simple command from God. God provided the light.

That leads me to this question: Are you living in a physical, mental, or spiritual "black hole"? Are you so imprisoned by destructive health habits, bitterness, shame, anger, lust, sadness, or a desire for revenge that the light of God's love can't even exist in your life? If so, the first step in God's Health Plan for you is the same step that God accomplished on the first day of Creation. He made light *possible* in the darkness. That's exactly what He will do in you if you'll give Him access to the dark corners of your heart. He wants to be the light of your life, the solution to a dark, stress-filled world.

Let me give you an illustration of what I'm talking about. A woman stands at the rain-splashed window of her house, gazing out at a storm. Her husband and children, on their way home from an outing, are an hour overdue. Thunder rattles the windows, lightning flashes, and the woman's body trembles with fear. She hasn't eaten supper, she can't relax, her head throbs, and her stomach is in knots from worry.

Then she sees the lights of the car in the driveway and the smiling, laughing faces of her children. Her husband waves apologetically as he guides the automobile into the garage. In that instant, the woman realizes that . . . she's hungry! Her heart returns to its normal rhythm. No more stomachache. No more pounding head. No more worry. Her family is safe, and she feels great joy and relief flooding her entire body. This is the way she's supposed to feel.

That's what happens when the light of God's love enters a darkened life. We begin to experience how we were designed to feel. We begin to be aware of destructive health habits needing to be set aside. We are able to offer forgiveness to others, and anger can begin to change into acceptance. When God's love illuminates a life, the transformation can begin.

A Two-Edged Sword

I must add, though, that this light of God's love is a two-edged sword, because many times, things long hidden begin to become painfully evident. Have you ever aimed the beam of a flashlight under your bed? If you haven't, you might want to prepare yourself for a shock. You may find stuff under there that you haven't seen since Carter was president. Light reveals much—sometimes more than you'd prefer to see. But you've got to know what's been making you sick before you can find healing. The light of truth will help you open your eyes and see.

Once God has taken up residence in your heart and you've determined to activate His Health Plan in your life, it's time to get to work, removing anything in your environment that could contribute to your physical, mental, or spiritual illness. Out go the dirty magazines and books, the violent DVDs, the toxic chemicals under the kitchen sink, the sugar- and salt-laden processed foods with little or no nutritional value, the websites filled with images that pollute the mind, the music that encourages selfish thoughts and actions. With God's help—perhaps with the guidance of a trained Christian counselor, if necessary—you begin to work out the anger, resentment, and bitterness that have been poisoning you for years. The darkness is replaced by God's healing light.

Sometimes, what's needed most in our lives is simply the awareness of God's presence. My ten-year-old son, Jake, provided a wonderful example of this recently. One night he tiptoed into our bedroom saying that he'd had a scary dream. Then he snuggled up next to me, and that's where he remained until dawn. He didn't say a word. He just needed the touch and presence of his father. His darkness—the darkness of a ten-year-old boy who's had scary dreams—was chased away by the love he felt from me. A love I was more than happy to share.

During our lives, we, too, may experience "scary dreams." One of these might include a health challenge, even for those of us who do our best to follow God's Health Plan. Our overstressed bodies do eventually wear out. But we know where to find wonderful light, even when all else fails. We know of a power that can bring a world into being from utter emptiness. We know of a love that shines a light into the darkest corners of our lives and is able to make something wonderful out of nothing.

On the first day of Creation, God demonstrated that He is able to bring light to the darkest places. That's what He wants to do with each one of us today. He wants us to be aware of His constant presence.

DAY 2—BREATHING LESSONS

Then God said, "Let there be a space between
the waters, to separate the waters of the heavens
from the waters of the earth." And that is what
happened. God made this space to separate the
waters of the earth from the waters of the
heavens. God called the space "sky."
And evening passed and morning came,
marking the second day.

—Genesis 1:6-8

Anyone who has ever taken an ocean voyage knows what the result of day two of Creation week looked like. All the voyager can see is a wide stretch of ocean extending to the horizon. Above that, sky; and hovering over it all, float white, billowing clouds made up of water—water separated from water, with air in between.

So how does this second day of Creation play into God's Health Plan for our lives? The answer is obvious, but all too often in the twenty-first century, the fundamentals of life are overlooked in favor of the latest trends in technology. It makes perfect sense that after giving us light to take away darkness, God would give water and air, key ingredients for our survival and also key components needed for health and the treatment of disease. Lacking just one of the two, we die.

I explained to David, "When you had a heart attack and went to the emergency room, what did they do first? They hooked you up to oxygen and started an IV so they could give you fluids."

"No problem," I can hear you saying. "I breathe all the time. As for water, I make sure I don't go thirsty by drinking plenty of liquids."

There's just one problem. Sure, we breathe—we pull air into our bodies and let it out. But what else besides oxygen is coming in with each of those breaths? And as for the liquids we consume each day, just how much of what we drink is actually water?

Life and Breath

Breathing is a way to change our chemistry. Just try holding your breath for a period of time, and you will notice some very definite changes taking place in you. When you breathe, you introduce oxygen into your entire system. Holding your breath can lower your oxygen levels and raise your carbon dioxide levels. Breathing fast can lower the carbon dioxide levels. Breathing either too slowly or too rapidly can affect the acid-base balance in the body. My point, in case you missed it, is that breathing is important. In Genesis 2:7 we read that God created Adam and "breathed the breath of life into the man's nostrils, and the man became a living person." Life and breath go together.

The effect of oxygen in us is profound. Our tissues need oxygen for survival. Have you ever wondered why you usually feel so good, so alive, while walking along a beach? The ocean is a veritable oxygen factory, releasing copious amounts of this precious element into the atmosphere from its submerged vegetation. We breathe in the oxygen-rich air and feel wonderful!

However, catching a good breath of air, which draws in the needed amount of oxygen, is getting a little more challenging these days. Stress can alter the way we breathe. When our bodies are under stress, we breathe more quickly and less deeply. This might be advantageous if we are in a fight for our lives—or when our bodies are responding to some acute *and temporary* situation. But stressful breathing for extended periods of time is damaging. Long-term stress means long-term lack of sufficient oxygen.

Then there's sleep apnea.

Martin ventured into my office a few years ago. He easily weighed five hundred pounds and stood only five feet eight inches tall. He was not happy about the state of his health, but he didn't know where to begin to turn things around. Depression had set in as he struggled with diabetes, high blood pressure, fatigue, headaches, and a litany of joint pains. Martin couldn't walk across the room without getting short of breath and running his heart rate up to 140 beats a minute. Life had turned into a real struggle for this thirty-nine-year-old. He'd never planned for this to happen, but one thing had led to another and . . . you get the picture. In addition, Martin's fifteen prescription medications were causing many side effects.

One of Martin's challenges was an ailment known as sleep apnea. This is a condition in which one doesn't get enough oxygen at night. Lack of oxygen means a lack of sound sleep, which results in a lack of tissue renewal. The whole body becomes stressed. Martin had been stressed by this condition for a third of his life. Can you imagine going under water, holding your breath as long as possible, and then coming up for breath? This was essentially what Martin was doing eight hours a day. Sleep apnea alone could explain the high blood pressure, headaches, fatigue, and palpitations he was experiencing. Martin needed help.

I explained the acute treatment for sleep apnea—the sleep mask to force oxygen into his lungs, and possible surgery, if indicated, to help open a blocked airway. However, as you'll continue to discover throughout this book, acute care addresses only the symptoms, not necessarily the causes of those symptoms. I needed to offer more. Martin was searching for a new approach, a hint of hope, and the ability to love himself back to health.

Does this sound familiar? Isn't that what we all need when facing seemingly insurmountable health problems? We often ask ourselves, *Is traditional medicine the way to go? Is there something more? Where are the answers for which I'm searching?*

Martin began with a common request: "Dr. Marcum, can't you just give me a pill to make me feel better?" I explained to him that the easiest thing in the world for me to do would be to prescribe yet another medication—number sixteen in his case—but that would not solve the underlying problem. We needed to go a step further. We needed to be honest. And I knew honesty had to be wrapped in love. I wasn't just dealing with a symptom. I was dealing with a living, breathing person. The truth was that Martin's problem was his weight and the behaviors that led to the weight.

I'm ashamed to admit it, but money and selfishness greatly influence the treatment of disease these days. There are many people making money from those who are sick. The cigarette industry, fast-food industry, health insurance industry, hospitals, producers of medical supplies, government, drug companies, and—yes—even physicians profit from people's suffering. The more patients suffer, the more others in these industries and professions stand to profit. For instance, much more money is made from a bypass surgery or from dispensing medications than from preventing a problem or dealing with the stress that will lead to problems down the road. Don't misunderstand me: I believe in and practice modern medicine. But there are often better solutions than a pill and a bill for every ill.

As I explained this to Martin, I could see him gaining interest and, more important, hope. He needed to lose weight. He needed to make some major changes to his lifestyle. He needed to return to God's Health Plan. I told him that sometimes the best medicine is no medicine. That's right. Sometimes the best way to heal a body is to get out of the way and let the incredible healing powers God placed in it do their own thing, unencumbered by drugs. We enact the prescriptions given at Creation.

This may be hard for our society to swallow when we spend one in six dollars on health care. But the truth is, chronic illness is not caused by a lack of pharmaceuticals. Breaking the divine laws of health is the real culprit. God created air for an important reason. Martin was robbing himself of this vital element by allowing himself to become obese. Obesity was causing a physical blockage of his airway when he was lying down. But if he were to lose weight, he would breathe better, and healing sleep would be restored. The answer to Martin's sleep apnea wasn't to be found in a bottle of pills. It was to be found at the dinner table.

That day my patient left my office with a renewed determination and a set of suggestions for curbing his appetite for unhealthy foods.

Relaxing Breaths

Breathing not only brings oxygen into the body, it can also help to relax the body. When you feel under stress, change your chemistry! Begin taking slow, deep breaths through the nose.

Hold for a few seconds and then exhale. You'll sense your body beginning to relax. This type of breathing is especially useful at night when you're preparing to rest, as this relaxes the body while enhancing oxygen delivery to the tissues.

A hundred years ago, lack of oxygen wasn't really that much of an issue. Physical work like plowing a field or building a barn provided that type of deep-breathing healing automatically. Walking instead of driving offered the same benefit. But as the world changed, so did our breathing patterns. We need to get back to the basics of our bodily chemistry, and nothing is more basic than breathing.

Right now, if you happen to be in a clean-air environment, I want you to take a few slow, deliberate deep breaths. Draw the air in through your nose. Hold it for five to ten seconds, then blow it out completely through your mouth. Now repeat. And then repeat again. See? Don't you feel more relaxed? That influx of oxygen just slowed your heart rate, lowered your blood pressure, and made your tissues very, very happy. No pill required.

The Challenge

Breathing in enough oxygen shouldn't be a problem for many of us. But some may face a challenge or two in this area. More and more homes and offices are tightly sealed to save energy costs. Unfortunately, that results in poor ventilation and the accumulation of indoor air pollutants. Formaldehyde, for example, seeps from certain wood products. Various fumes escape carpets, copy machines, upholstery, and cleaning products. Carbon monoxide and nitrogen dioxide—two poisonous gases—rise unseen from gas, oil, or coal furnaces, ranges, fireplaces, and heaters. Mix in a good dose of dust, mites, molds and fungi, ozone, lead, asbestos, pesticide residues, and a dash of radon gas and, well, suddenly all that air we breathe begins to take on a rather sinister character.

Yet how many warning labels do you see on synthetic household items or hanging over the door of your place of business?

In some areas, outside air may not be much of an improvement. Diesel fumes, factory pollutants spewing into the atmosphere, and even your neighbor mowing his postage-stamp-size lawn with a twenty-four-horsepower riding mower aren't exactly helping the situation. Do you see warnings printed on the sides of trucks or fastened on the steering wheels of riding mowers?

What are some of the results of breathing pollutant-laden air? Burning eyes, sore throats, coughing, itching, headaches, sluggishness, nausea, dizziness, feelings of exhaustion, and depression—the very types of symptoms that millions take to their doctors in order to get that "magic" and usually costly pill to address the problem.

Suddenly, enjoying all that clean air brought into existence on the second day of Creation seems like an impossible dream. How can we take advantage of this powerful element of God's Health Plan for our lives?

Here are some suggestions:

- First, ban all smoking indoors and out. Even secondhand smoke contains hundreds of harmful chemicals.
- Make sure your gas, oil, kerosene, and coal-burning heaters and appliances are well vented.
- Keep air ducts and heating and air-conditioning filters well maintained. Make sure your chimneys are open and in good repair.
- Finally—and this is so simple and important—keep fresh air coming into your home or office by opening a window if possible. Even in the dead of winter, open a window just a crack to allow clean, fresh air access to your home or office.

Breathe deeply of God's fresh air every day, and keep a good supply of oxygen coursing through your body with regular exercise. Remember, God created the sky for a reason.

The Water of Life

The second element of God's Health Plan that showed up on that second day of Creation was water. Not soda. Not milk. Not even fruit juice. Water!

I recently read a report from Loma Linda University. It had to do with this amazing liquid.

It's common knowledge that not drinking enough water has been linked to such ailments as constipation, kidney stones, overeating, and dry eyes, mouth, and skin. This new study, published in the *American Journal of Epidemiology*, showed that drinking high amounts of plain water is as important as exercise, diet, or not smoking in preventing coronary heart disease.

While that bit of information was surprising enough, what caught my eye was the word *plain* next to the word *water*. According to the study, neither total fluid intake nor intake of other fluids combined, showed this reduced risk. Coffee, soda, milk, and caffeinated drinks offered no significant heart benefits. In fact, these types of fluids draw water *from* the blood, because they can't be absorbed until their concentration is similar to that of the blood. *Plain* water, however, is absorbed immediately and quickly hydrates the system, thinning the blood and thus reducing the risk of clots that can lead to a heart attack.

The study concluded with these words: "Because drinking more plain water is a simple lifestyle change that anybody can do, this practice has the potential of saving tens of thousands of lives each year with minimal cost."

Listen to how Jesus, speaking to a woman at a well, described His presence in a person's life: "Those who drink the water I give will never be thirsty again. It becomes a fresh, bubbling spring within them, giving them eternal life" (John 4:14). God's love does the same thing to a person's spiritual life that water does for his or her physical life.

Divine Dilution

After I read the Loma Linda study, a dark thought crossed my mind concerning my spiritual health. How often do I "dilute" my heavenly Father? How often do I accept the God of my church or the God of my favorite sermon CD or the God of the latest bestseller as my Savior? How often do I add a little extra ingredient to my relationship with Him that actually does nothing to enhance His power in my life? All these things do is make God "taste" better in my mind or make Him "blend" more unobtrusively with my appetite for sin.

I'm determined to build my relationship with the "plain" God I find when I close my eyes in prayer or walk in the shaded solitude of a forest. As a matter of fact, if enough of you will join me, we'll create our own "scientific" study that will end with these words: "Because worshiping the 'plain' God is a simple lifestyle change that anybody can do, this practice has the potential of saving tens of thousands of souls each year with minimal cost."

God's Health Plan includes *plain* water—not the messed-with liquid we find in colorful bottles and cans at the grocery store. It's not fruit juices, vegetable mixtures, or all-natural smoothies—healthy enough in their own right—that God created on that second day. No, He made water—plain and simple. Unfortunately, many of us bypass that no-calories wonder on a regular basis.

It's common knowledge in the medical community that a vast majority of Americans are suffering from dehydration. In fact, it is estimated that up to 70 percent of us do not hydrate ourselves adequately. It is not fun to walk in a hot desert. It causes the stress chemistry to be activated. Imagine, in a land where clean water is as close as our kitchen sinks, we're robbing our bodies of one of the most important requirements for a healthy life.

Water lubricates the body parts, flushes out impurities, protects us from diseases, and keeps us going when others fade. As a matter of fact, Africans have another name for this liquid, and we should keep it in mind. In their countries, water is simply called "life."

How much water should you drink? Here's a simple rule to follow. The average adult body loses around ten to twelve cups of water a day through the skin, lungs, urine, and feces. A whole-foods, plant-based diet provides up to four cups of water, leaving us eight cups short. This should be added to our systems using plain, un-messed-with water filtered straight from the tap or well. Another suggestion is to divide your body weight by two. The result tells you approximately how many ounces of water a healthy person needs each day.

Do you want a great start to your day? Drink a glass of room-temperature water right after you get up, and then again in midmorning. Do you want to keep going and going and going? Enjoy another glass of water in midafternoon and again in early evening. And at all times, follow this simple rule: if you're thirsty, drink *water*.

The real reason we are becoming more sick as a society is that we are losing sight of what God had in mind for keeping us healthy when He created us. He created air and water on day two for an important reason. We have a tendency to turn away from the simple yet powerful truths He gave us at the beginning and to focus our attention on science and technology to heal our ills. It's so important that we return to the basics of what the Creator provided for us as we work to regain and maintain optimum health.

As David and I finished discussing these verses and concepts, David agreed that before that day he had never thought of water and air as treatments that were as important as his prescriptions. He was becoming eager to learn. He was discovering truth. He began to hear God's Spirit speaking to his heart. And he could hardly wait for day three.

9

DAY 3—HEALTH ON SOLID GROUND

THEN GOD SAID, "LET THE WATERS BENEATH THE SKY
FLOW TOGETHER INTO ONE PLACE, SO DRY GROUND MAY
APPEAR." AND THAT IS WHAT HAPPENED. GOD CALLED THE
DRY GROUND "LAND" AND THE WATERS "SEAS." AND GOD
SAW THAT IT WAS GOOD. THEN GOD SAID, "LET THE LAND
SPROUT WITH VEGETATION—EVERY SORT OF SEED-BEARING
PLANT, AND TREES THAT GROW SEED-BEARING FRUIT.
THESE SEEDS WILL THEN PRODUCE THE KINDS OF PLANTS
AND TREES FROM WHICH THEY CAME." AND THAT IS WHAT
HAPPENED. . . . AND EVENING PASSED AND MORNING CAME,
MARKING THE THIRD DAY.

—GENESIS 1:9-11, 13

WHAT IF I TOLD you that scientists had unearthed something
that would greatly lower or, in some cases, completely remove
your risk of cancer, heart disease, and diabetes? Interested? Well,
that amazing breakthrough is available today—not at the drugstore, but at your local *grocery* store.

I recently heard a story from an international development
and relief agency. It seems that in Mongolia, winters had been
especially severe—so severe that many of the animals that the
people used for food had died. The good folk at the agency knew
that if something was not done right away, many Mongolians

would perish from starvation. Their food source was dying in the cold.

So they rolled up their sleeves and got to work, teaching people how to grow vegetable gardens using weather-resistant seeds, proper irrigation, and nonchemical fertilizers. Soon neat, green rows of growing vegetables could be seen in garden plots large and small throughout the country. Little by little, the diet of thousands of Mongolians changed from being *animal* based to being *plant* based.

As hoped, starvation was averted. The people who had gardens survived very well and were even able to help their neighbors stay alive. After the agency showed them how to build economical storage buildings, communities began enjoying sufficient supplies of garden-grown food year-round.

But that's not the end of the story. When representatives followed up with those who had adopted the new plant-based diet, they learned something interesting. Children who ate their veggies instead of meat suffered from fewer colds and other illnesses. Adults enjoyed more energy and better health, bypassing many of the sicknesses sweeping the country. They were not only alive; they were alive *and well*. All they had done was alter their diet to be plant based.

This really shouldn't surprise us. After all, what those Mongolians had unknowingly done was adopt a powerful component of God's Health Plan—a plan He created right along with the rest of this earth.

At the end of the third day of Creation week, the Creator left behind not a world "formless and empty," as it had been before. No, He left a world of land, sea, vegetation, and sky. In other words, God had created a farm! But there was one problem. As any schoolchild knows, plants need more than air and water to grow. They need something else. They need sunlight.

That is why the very next day, God said, "'Let lights appear in the sky to separate the day from the night. . . .' God made two great lights—the larger one to govern the day, and the smaller one to govern the night" (Genesis 1:14, 16).

On that fourth day, this world fairly exploded with plant life after the sun appeared. Have you ever seen those time-lapse movies of flowers opening up or vines growing along stone walls? In those amazing film clips, days and weeks are compressed into mere seconds. That is what it may have looked like when the plants created on day three found themselves staring up at day four's sun. It must've been awesome!

We'll explore the powerful health-building properties of the sun in our next chapter. But just for a moment, let's move forward a few days to when God is standing with Adam and Eve in their new garden home. The Creator's arm sweeps over the verdant growth surrounding them, indicating the fruit-heavy trees and produce-laden plants. With a satisfied smile, He turns to the happy couple. "Look! I have given you every seed-bearing plant throughout the earth," He tells them in Genesis 1:29, "and all the fruit trees for your food."

And that brings us back to the Mongolians. When they changed their diet to the foods God originally intended for humankind to eat, their health improved. Their minds became clearer; their energy levels increased. We shouldn't be surprised. Instead, we should praise God that the Creator's Health Plan is still changing lives today. As David and I continued to learn, I wanted to introduce him to yet another component of the original plan.

Why Plants?

So what's so special about fruits and vegetables? What do they have that animal products—foods made from animal flesh—don't have? Actually, the more relevant question is, What do fruits and vegetables *not* have that animal-based products contain?

In the first comprehensive *Surgeon General's Report on Nutrition and Health (1985)*, former surgeon general Dr. C. Everett Koop stated that the Western diet was a major contributor to heart disease, cancer, and stroke. He confirmed that saturated fat and cholesterol found in abundance in animal protein of all kinds were the main culprits. He pointed out that these foods were usually eaten at the expense of selections rich in complex carbohydrates, such as whole grains, legumes, and vegetables.

In *Health Power: Health by Choice, Not Chance* (Review and Herald 2001), epidemiologist Hans Diehl states, "The risk for cancer of the prostate, breast, and colon is three to four times higher for people who consume meat, eggs, and dairy products on a daily basis when compared to those who eat them sparingly or not at all. In addition, vegetarian women have stronger bones and fewer fractures, and they lose less bone as they age" (p. 183).

To underscore his point, Dr. Diehl, the founder/director of CHIP (Coronary Health Improvement Project), adds that the results of research centered on long-lived vegetarians like the Hunzas of Pakistan, who are healthy and active into advanced age, contrast sharply with the short life spans and increased disease rates of traditional Eskimos, who depend largely on what they catch in the sea or hunt on the frozen tundra.

Health studies and statistics are one thing. But what do your eyes tell you when you walk through any mall in America or take part in any social gathering? Do we look healthy to you? Why are drugstore shelves lined with increasingly powerful headache and stomachache medications? Why are obesity and diabetes rates soaring? Why are teenagers experiencing health problems that just a few years ago stalked only the elderly? The answer is diet. We're eating the wrong foods at the wrong times in the wrong amounts. And we are paying a terrible price for doing so.

God's Health Plan was complete at the end of Creation week. Adam and Eve needed nothing else—no wonder drugs, no pills or powders, no fat-filled fast foods, no dairy products, no meat dishes, no heavily refined foods in convenient take-home packaging. All they needed was right there before them in the Garden.

Modern Messages

Epidemiologist Dr. T. Colin Campbell in his groundbreaking book *The China Study* (BenBella Books 2004) took a balanced, scientific look at the world's food sources and concluded that a plant-based diet is the only way to go. Here's how he summed up his many years of study and research in the field of nutrition and health:

> Almost all of us in the United States will die of diseases of affluence. In our China Study, we saw that nutrition has a very strong effect on these diseases. Plant-based foods are linked to lower blood cholesterol; animal-based foods are linked to higher blood cholesterol. Animal-based foods are linked to higher breast cancer rates; plant-based foods are linked to lower rates. Fiber and antioxidants from plants are linked to a lower risk of cancers of the digestive tract. Plant-based diets and active lifestyles result in a healthy weight, yet permit people to become big and strong. . . . From the labs of Virginia Tech and Cornell University to the far reaches of China, it seemed that science was painting a clear, consistent picture: we can minimize our risk of contracting deadly diseases just by eating the right food. (p. 105)

Why don't we hear more about this? The answer is heart-breaking. It's all about the money. The media—and the advertisers who support the media—control our thoughts. And, as I've said before, there is more money to be made by making and keeping us sick than by helping us get well. I'm not surprised by Dr. Campbell's conclusion based on his decades of research. After all, the diet he found to be the most healthful was the very diet God placed before Adam and Eve in Eden: fruits, vegetables, nuts, grains, and plain water. No diet could be better.

Even in the book of Daniel, we see this point driven home. When offered the "affluence" diet of the king—a diet rich in animal protein, which the poor people in the kingdom could not afford—Daniel and his friends made a request: "Daniel was determined not to defile himself by eating the food and wine given to them by the king. He asked the chief of staff for permission not to eat these unacceptable foods. Now God had given the chief of staff both respect and affection for Daniel. But he responded, 'I am afraid of my lord the king, who has ordered that you eat this food and wine. If you become pale and thin compared to the other youths your age, I am afraid the king will have me beheaded'" (Daniel 1:8-10).

Does this sound familiar? "You need animal protein to grow big and strong!" Advertisers shout from television sets and magazine pages. "Real men eat beef" and "Milk builds strong bones." We see beer manufacturers sponsoring sporting events, and the tobacco industry wants us to believe that dumping two hundred plus poisons into our lungs is "cool." But Daniel had a very different vision—one based not on the media but on his Maker: "Daniel spoke with the attendant who had been appointed by the chief of staff to look after Daniel, Hananiah, Mishael, and Azariah. 'Please test us for ten days on a diet of vegetables and water,' Daniel said. 'At the end of the ten days, see how we look compared to the other young men who are eating the king's food. Then make your decision in light of what you see.' The attendant agreed to Daniel's suggestion and tested them for ten days" (1:11-14).

There was a lot at stake here, to say nothing of the chief of staff's head! So how did this ancient health study play out? We find the results starting in verse 15: "At the end of the ten days, Daniel and his three friends looked healthier and better nourished than the young men who had been eating the food assigned by the king. So after that, the attendant fed them only vegetables instead. . . . When the training period ordered by the king was completed, the chief of staff brought all the young men to King Nebuchadnezzar. The king talked with them, and no one impressed him as much as Daniel, Hananiah, Mishael, and Azariah. So they entered the royal service. Whenever the king consulted them in any matter requiring wisdom and balanced judgment, he found them ten times more capable than any of the magicians and enchanters in his entire kingdom" (1:15-16, 18-20).

I don't know about you, but I think there's a definite message here for our public education system. Want smart kids? Feed them the right foods!

Acute Care

Modern medicine is great at acute care. Break a leg? We're there. Fighting an infectious disease? We're ready. Suffered a serious injury? Bring it on. But we are not all that effective when it comes to dealing with the effects of too many toxins, a sparseness of nutrients in many acres of overworked soil, and massive amounts of chemicals in our food, water, and air. Just as in Daniel's time, some of us can't even think right. The solution today—as it was then—is to boost our intake of needed nutrients by selecting organic foods, detoxifying our bodies, and getting back to the Creator's original Health Plan.

Keep in mind that even "good foods" can be bad if they are

loaded with chemicals used to color, flavor, and preserve them. Read labels. If you can't pronounce an ingredient in the list, you probably can't digest it either. Such additives and "enhancers" create chronic stress on our systems. We are now hearing about chemicals being leached from food storage containers and eventually entering our bodies. Chemicals from plastic, including bisphenol A, can simulate our hormonal system and travel from cell to cell, causing damage. These foreign estrogens, called xenoestrogens, do not belong in our bodies and can be very destructive to young people as they grow and develop, especially individuals with susceptible DNA.

These xenoestrogens have been found in plastics, pesticides, cosmetics, cleaners, and a host of other products. And we wonder why we're experiencing lower fertility rates, more prostate cancer, more birth defects, autism, and other conditions never seen before to this degree.

Reports in the *Journal of the American Medical Association* (JAMA 2008:300[11]:1303–1310) have linked these chemicals with increased risk of cardiovascular disease, diabetes, and liver abnormalities. Recently, chemicals called phthalates, also found in plastics, have been shown to damage the reproductive system and have been linked to cancer. And just think—only a few years ago, six billion pounds of bisphenol A (BPA) were produced.

Thanks to the information age, knowledge, as well as deception, gets around fast. But there's another problem facing even those of us who are trying to follow God's original diet.

Mutant Munchies

Genetically modified foods are everywhere in our food supply. What is genetic modification? Genetic material with desired characteristics from a different species is inserted into the DNA of a plant or animal. For instance, genetic material is inserted in corn or cotton to enable it to make its own pesticide. Such a process is occurring with increasing frequency in our food supply, and we don't really understand the long-term implications.

Toxic and allergic reactions have already been documented. Genetic-modification technology is being used not only in our food supply but also in vaccines and drugs. Common sense indicates there is a very good chance that this will put stress on our bodies and affect our health.

"But don't worry," says the medical profession. "We probably have a medication to mask the symptoms for a while."

Just to put this into perspective and provide a tiny peek into the profits waiting to be made by the drug companies and health care facilities, here are a few of the diseases associated with chronic stress on a system: headaches, depression, anxiety, insomnia, Alzheimer's disease, panic disorders, eating disorders, obesity and subsequent health problems, diabetes, heart attacks, hypertension, infections because of weak immune systems, osteoporosis, ulcers, sexual dysfunction, acid reflux, irritable bowel syndrome, fibromyalgia, acne, psoriasis, eczema, shingles, arthritis, multiple sclerosis, lupus, chronic muscle and joint pain, and memory loss. Are you beginning to see the broader picture here?

You Are What You Eat

Mrs. Brown is known for her great Southern biscuits. I have tasted them, and they are delicious! But Mrs. Brown, now in her late fifties, grew up eating sugarcoated cereal and fast food. As an adult, she continued eating sugarcoated cereal in the morning, fast food during lunch break, and then a large meal at night—sometimes topped off with a bowl of ice cream. After dinner, she usually watched television or surfed the Internet until bedtime.

I saw Mrs. Brown in the office a few months ago. Her main

complaints were a feeling of fatigue and frequent trips to the bathroom. Testing revealed diabetes, high cholesterol, and hypertension. Most of these problems could be attributed to nutrition.

The saying "You are what you eat" has been passed down through many years. There's a lot of truth in the statement. Many, especially those in fast-paced industrialized and highly technological societies, have similar diets. Our culture promotes fast food, frozen food, salty food, fried food, high-caloric food, processed food, and too much food. This type of promotion is causing incredible amounts of suffering. Yes, this might be the more convenient way to eat, but it's totally messing up our chemistry and putting stress on our systems. We are being deceived into thinking we must follow the status quo and eat the way we always have, the way we were taught, or the foods we see in advertising.

I, like most of us, have struggled with nutrition. Medical schools barely touch on the subject. Most hospitals fail to emphasize nutrition as treatment. And to further stir the waters, there seems to be a new nutrition or diet book out every week. Many people are overwhelmed and confused by the wide variety of voices shouting out their messages.

However, two important themes seem to remain consistent in all of modern nutritional literature: (1) you are what you eat, and (2) eating is a habit.

When I first started practicing medicine many years ago, I was very idealistic and encouraged my patients to eat perfectly. I remember one old-timer who looked over at me from his perch on the examination table. "Doc," he said, "I'd rather die than give up my fried 'taters.'"

Through the years, I have tried to develop a more realistic, commonsense approach to nutrition. I try to teach my patients what God designed us to eat, but I also recognize that eating habits developed in childhood make up a big part of who we are.

This entire book has been built on biblical teachings, on getting back to the original owner's manual outlined in Eden. I ask my patients, "What does God teach us about nutrition?" Then I show them that often overlooked verse in Genesis that puts all questions to rest. God, speaking to Adam and Eve said, "Look! I have given you every seed-bearing plant throughout the earth and all the fruit trees for your food" (Genesis 1:29). Pretty straightforward, isn't it?

Fuel

The story is told of a man who bought a brand-new car and proudly drove it home from the dealer. But in just a few weeks, his pride and joy began to develop problems. It backfired a lot, smoked terribly, and was hard to start. The engine knocked continually and had very little power to climb the smallest hill.

In a huff, the man jerked and backfired his way to the dealer, where he demanded his money back. "You sold me a lemon!" he said angrily.

The dealer walked around the car and peered under the hood at the overheated engine. "I don't understand," he said. "People love this particular model." Turning to the irate customer, he asked, "You are keeping oil and gasoline in it, aren't you?"

The man lifted his chin. "I put the best diesel fuel in it each and every week."

Opening the car's owner's manual, the dealer pointed to a notation on page 1. "Sir," he said, "this car was designed to run on regular, unleaded fuel, not diesel. That's what's causing *all* the problems. You've been putting the wrong fuel into the tank."

Of course, this raises the question, What fuel are we putting into our bodies? Our owner's manual, written by our Designer, has made it more than clear that we were made to run on certain foods. He pointed them out, one by one, to Adam and Eve. He makes them available to us today in our grocery stores. Even science is showing the value of a plant-based diet consisting of fresh fruits, vegetables, nuts, and grains. The antioxidants and phytochemicals contained in these "fuels" promote health, fight inflammation, and give us boundless energy, while diets high in fat—especially the trans-saturated fats found in most fast foods—damage our sometimes delicate systems.

The animals people eat are another major issue. They have their own set of health problems, and to get them to market faster, many producers give them chemicals to make them grow at an accelerated rate. These health problems and powerful chemicals are passed on to us when we eat their meat or drink their milk. To put it simply, it's the wrong fuel, and it causes a cascade of problems within our bodies.

The Shopping Trip

I'm not much of a shopper. I'm just not that crazy about lugging bulging bags between specialty shops and superstores. But there is one type of shopping I easily tolerate—*grocery* shopping. Just give me a list of foods the Marcum household needs and turn me loose!

I always head straight for the produce section of our favorite grocery store. Then I stop and smile, imagining Adam and Eve standing in their garden looking over many of the same types of fruits, vegetables, grains, nuts, and legumes that I see. What a rainbow of colors meets my eye as I pick out my favorite fruits, dig through the display of vegetables, load up my cart with dried beans for the slow cooker, choose the freshest whole-grain breads and cereals, and gather enough soy or rice milk to see us through the coming week. I proudly stand in line at the checkout counter as those around me study my collection with a touch of knowing in their eyes.

Then all week, when I sit down to meals, I find great satisfaction in the fact that no animal had to suffer and pay the supreme sacrifice so I could fill my hungry stomach. Eating what God originally intended for me to eat is not only physically healthful but also has a positive impact on my mental and spiritual well-being.

The Whole Truth

What's the best way to eat the foods highlighted in God's Health Plan? One word: *whole*. That means there is nothing missing. Everything that's supposed to be in it is there. The benefits are far reaching. Diabetics, for instance, have for many years been instructed to stay away from sugars. Fruit juices are no-nos. But studies are revealing that if diabetics eat the *whole* fruit—complete with fiber—their bodies respond more slowly and evenly to the natural sugars the fruit contains, and no damage is done.

God in His infinite wisdom created the foods that grow in the ground or hang from the trees in such a way that we receive their full load of nutrition only when we eat them whole. All those powerful, cancer-fighting antioxidants, minerals, vitamins, and other healing nutrients find their way into our bodies via the fiber, juices, and protective coverings of those foods. *Whole* grains. *Whole* fruits. *Whole* vegetables—food as God intended.

When we start isolating the elements in foods and eating them far removed from their original form, we weaken their potential. That's what "refining" does—it separates elements into individual products. Sugarcane becomes table sugar. Whole-wheat flour ends up as white flour. Fruits get squeezed into fruit juices. And, though we often peel, the lowly potato is best served with its skin, even when mashed.

Healthy Love

Before we leave this amazing third day of Creation, I want to share a thought with you. As we are discovering in the chapters of this book, it takes more than good food choices to build and maintain optimum health. Good health is also related to the way we live and to what lives in our hearts. So often I hear people dwelling only on the food aspect. Eat this. Don't eat that. Now don't get me wrong; food is very important to health. Unfortunately, I have seen some people getting angry, judgmental, or even depressed over their diets. These emotions are probably more dangerous than the unhealthy food they are telling everyone to avoid.

Sound bodies require healthy thoughts, commonsense exercise, focused worship, and thankful, loving hearts. The Holy Spirit—when He has access to our minds—will lovingly lead us to physical health at our own speed and through avenues we trust. When we come to God with our shortcomings, He will give us the power to build and maintain optimum spiritual health as well. He doesn't want us to get down on others, or on ourselves.

When I see people being judgmental or overreacting about any one aspect of their personal health plans, I'm concerned. Please, don't make healthy habits into gods. Don't worship at the throne of food, exercise, perfect lab numbers, ideal weight, or other health details. Worship the God who created you, and reflect His loving nature to those with whom you come in contact.

What a wonderful Creator God! He formed us. He knows us inside and out. And He has made it possible for all—even hungry Mongolians—to enjoy the health benefits of eating the diet He prepared for us. When we blend heavenly love with the Eden diet, that's enough to make anyone healthy and happy.

Getting Real

Since the stress of eating the wrong things (foods devoid of nutritional value and high in saturated fats, salt, and sugar) is such a major component of disease, I would like to offer a practical eating plan. It has been proven time and time again that if people make small changes, three things happen: they start to feel better, they save money, and they enjoy more control over their health.

If you happen to be a jogger, you will know exactly what I'm talking about. You start out your jog tired from the day's work, depressed over that run-in with your spouse, and feeling totally worthless. But a funny thing happens around block three. Something begins to change in your psyche. You find yourself strangely energized, even though you are expending energy. Your subconscious kicks in with a few suggestions on how to reconnect with the one you love, and your sense of self-worth begins to creep back up again. The more you run, the more you want to run, because it feels so good. You're experiencing a cascade of chemical changes in your body—changes that are reviving your mind, body, and spirit.

That is exactly what it's like when you begin making slow but steady nutritional adjustments. The "commonsense light" begins to turn on in your awakening brain. Suddenly, you sense the danger in eating fatty foods as your doctor has warned that fat can build up in your arteries. If you are overweight, the thought that you should consume fewer calories begins to really sink in. If high blood pressure is a problem, you are suddenly shocked at the high sodium numbers shouting at you from food labels. Like disease, health is self-perpetuating. There is no middle ground. Your lifestyle is either heading you for the hospital or for a healthier future.

Eat Smart

So how do you eat smart? Consider these suggestions that can save not only your heart but also your life. If you eat French fries every day, you might start by eating them only once a week, and then maybe just on special occasions like a birthday. If you eat greasy hamburgers every day at lunch, you might want to start by choosing a "garden burger" as a meatless meal every other day and toss in a salad with a little fat-free dressing on the side. Hooked on colas? Substitute a sweet, tangy fruit juice 50 percent of the time, or best of all, learn to enjoy the simple taste of water. Gotta have that morning coffee with its dangerous load of caffeine? Become more sophisticated and start enjoying hot herbal teas instead. Just try not to look too smug when your coworkers see you drinking it.

Once you begin making these small changes, your body chemistry will start to improve, and you'll find yourself willing—dare I say eager—to make more changes because you feel much better.

When you eat can be just as important as what you eat. Many of my patients work all day, come home, eat a big meal composed mostly of highly processed foods, flop down on the couch, watch television, and then finish out the evening with a bowl of ice cream. I don't mean to gross you out, but when we fill our stomachs with food—any food—late in the evening, then go to bed, that load of nutrients kind of just sits there all night long. Not much digestion takes place while we sleep. It doesn't take much imagination to visualize what happens to organic material when it's stored for seven hours in a warm, moist place. Then, when we get up in the morning, we wonder why we feel so lousy, have absolutely no appetite, and have breath that smells like the family cat that crawled into the dirty clothes hamper and died. So here's what I recommend. Eat a much smaller meal as early in the evening as possible. Then you might want to head out for a short walk in the fresh air and burn off some of those calories.

Some people can make all the dietary changes I listed below at once and be totally happy about the change. They are probably in the minority. When I'm creating a treatment plan based on good nutrition, I try to individualize it, remembering that happiness is important too. The "I'm going to change my lifestyle" mentality must place its focus on what we *can* do, not on what we can't. We *can* eat healthier food. We *can* live longer. We *can* cut our doctor bills. We *can* have more energy. We *can* bypass most of the diseases plaguing modern society. We are not giving up food; we are simply changing our menus. In the great salad bar of life, we are choosing to load our plates with food that God created especially for our bodies.

Practical Suggestions

This is not intended to be a nutrition book, but I do want to offer some practical suggestions for improving your nutritional intake. I'll give it to you straight, based on endless scientific studies and on what I have seen work best in my patients:

1. **Eat a balanced diet with lots of fresh fruits, vegetables, nuts, whole grains, legumes, and seeds.** This would include soy, rice, beans, and whole-grain pastas. Fad diets can be harmful.
2. **Drink more water, and avoid soft drinks.** Stay away from anything that contains corn syrup.
3. **Avoid foods with a high fat content.** These are basically fried foods, meats, French fries, cheese, eggs, margarine and butter, ice cream, doughnuts, cookies, gravy, potato

chips, and so on. These are high in trans-saturated fats (trans fats), which cause all sorts of stress and chemical problems in the body.

4. **Sparingly use monounsaturated fats like olive oil and canola oil.** You might learn how to leave them out completely. The body doesn't process such fats. It stores them. I don't have to tell you where.

5. **Reduce salt intake by diminishing your use of table salt and processed foods.** Remember, too much salt can increase blood pressure, which can lead to cardiovascular disease, kidney disease, osteoporosis, and kidney stones. In fact, half the people on dialysis are there because of high blood pressure. Try Bragg Liquid Aminos instead of salt to enhance taste without loading your body down with sodium.

6. **Avoid eating *only* for pleasure.** Eat when you are hungry; stop when you are full. Eat smaller portions slowly. By the way, foods high in fiber (plant-based foods) send a clear "I'm full" signal to the brain, which switches off the hunger sensation at just the right moment. Nonfiber foods (animal products and highly processed foods) do not. Something to think about.

7. **Eat most of your calories in the morning.** Not hungry when you get up? Simply eat a smaller supper and nothing after seven in the evening. The chemical reactions that result from skipping breakfast make it very hard for you to make good food choices later in the day.

8. **Become a vegetarian.** Even most animals are vegetarians. When you eat meat, you're getting your calories secondhand. In addition, the diseases the animals might have, the steroids used to promote growth, and chemicals added to the animals' foods are passed on to you. Animal

products are also absolutely loaded with fat. "But I'll just eat fish or only organic animal products," many patients say. While this is certainly a step in the right direction, meat is meat, and we weren't designed to process it in any form.

9. **Avoid processed foods and the chemical additives found in them.** Here's a simple rule: look for packaged foods with the fewest ingredients. Again, if you can't pronounce an ingredient, you probably can't digest it.

10. **Eliminate caffeine and alcohol from your diet.** These are two powerful toxins that do much more harm than good.

11. **Be careful with supplements and herbs.** Take the time to learn about them from a reliable source. Some herbs interfere with cardiac medications. It's always best to get your nutritional needs from whole foods—foods as they were grown.

12. **Eat plenty of antioxidants.** These amazing micronutrients have the incredible ability to fight the development and spread of cancer cells. Where do we find these antioxidants? In plant-based foods like fruits and legumes.

13. **Find foods with omega-3, -6, -9 fatty acids—the healthy fats.** Again, choose plant-based foods—like flaxseeds for omega-3. Grind flaxseeds before adding them to your diet.

I hope you're not overwhelmed after reading the list. Instead, I hope you're encouraged. There *is* hope for you and your family. There *is* a plan you can follow to bypass the bypass, to reduce the risk of contracting cancer, to shield yourself from the diseases that are filling doctors' offices and hospital beds.

Choose a couple of items from the list and try to follow those suggestions for a month. I guarantee you will feel better. Once those become habits, pick another suggestion from the list and work on it as well. After all, you only have one body and one life to live. You are in charge of your choices. When it comes to lifestyle diseases, you decide how sick—or how healthy—you want to be.

Junk Money

The world wants you to eat poorly. There's a lot of money to be made when you eat "junk." There are deceptions at every turn. But eating the right foods can change your chemistry and act just like medications without the terrible side effects. Eating nutritionally devalued foods can cause stress and can be compared to slow poison.

Many of our modern-day medications are derived from plants. There are entrepreneurs who search the world for powerful chemicals in plants and foods that help our bodies. When they find them, they isolate these chemicals and try to market them to us as the latest and greatest miracle cure, which can be ours for just $19.95 plus shipping and handling. There's just one problem: isolating nutrients from their source removes them from the "delivery mechanism" God created for that nutrient. In isolation, these nutrients can sometimes become impotent or in some cases can be dangerous.

My friend Dr. T. Colin Campbell, in his book *The China Study*, calls this type of endeavor "scientific reductionism." Here is what he says: "As long as scientists study highly isolated chemicals and food components, and take the information out of context to make sweeping assumptions about complex diet and disease relationships, confusion will result. Misleading news headlines about this or that food chemical and this or that disease will be the norm" (p. 286).

Then Dr. Campbell concludes: "Scientific investigations of the effects of single nutrients on complex diseases have little or no meaning when the main dietary effect is due to the consumption of an extraordinary collection of nutrients and other substances found in whole foods" (p. 288).

Let me give you one example. Resveratrol is a phytochemical found in the skin of red grapes and other plants such as berries, plums, and peanuts. This chemical increases the activity of some sirtuin enzymes, thought to be involved in the regulation of aging. Dietary supplements containing resveratrol are now being widely promoted as antioxidants that can slow or prevent age-related illnesses.

Wow! Pop a pill and slow aging and disease. But guess what? Studies have shown that caloric restriction (eating less) also increases sirtuin activity and that a calorie-restricted diet delayed the onset of age-related diseases and extended the life spans of primates in the lab.

So why would anyone want to shell out big bucks to buy an isolated part of certain foods when simply going down to the grocery store and buying a nice bag of tasty red grapes, berries, plums, and peanuts does exactly the same things without having to enroll yourself in a worldwide scientific study of what happens to the human body when it is introduced to an isolated nutrient from a whole food? Why not just eat the chemical as God gave it to us in nature?

I have an uneasy feeling that as time goes by, we will begin hearing rumors of where that particular study is taking us. But are you hearing about studies that show the amazing health benefits of eating grapes, berries, plums, and peanuts? No. Why? Because unlike those isolated nutrients in pill form, the foods themselves are not moneymakers.

Let me give you some examples of foods with proven—under

the marketing radar—chemical benefits. Pomegranate juice and soy milk can lower prostate-specific antigen (PSA). Alzheimer's disease can be helped by the antioxidants found in blueberries, strawberries, and grapes. (These same antioxidants can also lower cholesterol and blood pressure.)

Turmeric and the vitamin D triggered in the body by exposure to sunlight can help fight breast cancer. Alpha omega fatty acids found in walnuts, almonds, flaxseed, and spinach can ease depression, lower cholesterol, and help nerve function.

Kelp can assist the thyroid. Oatmeal—or anything with fiber, such as almonds and walnuts, soy, and garlic—can lower cholesterol, thus decreasing the risk of cardiovascular disease. Beans, artichokes, chestnuts, carrots, onions, honey, pineapple, and almost any whole, plant-based food you can think of now have the science to prove their chemical benefits.

Indeed, the very food God gave us in the beginning is treatment for the disease states we have inherited and acquired. But are we rushing to the produce section of our grocery stores so we can fight these diseases? No. We're forming lines at the drugstore, hoping that the latest technological cure will keep us alive to see another day.

Why don't we hear God's Health Plan being shouted from the hilltops and televised with our favorite police drama? Because God is not an entrepreneur. He is simply a loving Savior who makes good health available to anyone who can chew and swallow.

Our society puts those who murder behind bars. Yet dangerous foods that are literally killing us are promoted and not condemned.

Don't be deceived. Don't make it harder than it needs to be. Use common sense. Science will never prove God wrong, because God is the One who created science. When making future food choices, ask God for help. Recall the words of the apostle Paul in Philippians 4:13: "I can do everything through Christ, who gives me strength."

We have covered quite a bit of ground as we've looked at day three of Creation. This same information gave my patient David a new appreciation for the kinds of foods he eats. He now realizes that the basic principles of nutrition were given at Creation. I hope you understand, as I have learned, that the real solution to the health care dilemma was given a very long time ago.

10

DAY 4—YOU'VE GOT RHYTHM

God said, "Let lights appear in the sky to separate
the day from the night. Let them be signs to
mark the seasons, days, and years. Let these lights
in the sky shine down on the earth." And that
is what happened. . . .
And evening passed and morning came,
marking the fourth day.

—Genesis 1:14-15, 19

When we next met, David was prepared and already knew
about the fourth day of Creation week. "Dr. Marcum, how in
the world does the fourth day relate to my health? I just can't see
how the sun and stars are a part of God's Health Plan." He was
reading his Bible. A relationship was forming. God was getting
through to him. I must admit, this was exciting to me.

Our earth is a solar-powered world, enjoying 98 percent of
its warmth from that bright, round orb that rises in the east and
sets in the west. That endless solar power lifts clouds, pushes the
wind, and generates photosynthesis in the plants that feed all
living things.

Sunlight also kills germs, boosts our spirits, and enhances our health in ways that are only now becoming known.

So, knowing all that, what do we do? We *hide* from the sun! We cover ourselves, shield our skin from the sun's rays, slather on chemicals designed to ensure that no UV particle worth its salt will get past our oily defenses. We wear hats, sunglasses, and long-sleeved shirts. We pull the curtains, close the shades, and light our world with artificial sources. The sun has become a boiling bogeyman trying to hunt us down and steal our health with its cancer-producing brilliance.

There's one problem. History does not record a single civilization dying off because the people allowed the sun to shine unencumbered on their cities and homes. Not one moldy, handwritten historical document hiding in a library somewhere includes these words: "The culture died because the people failed to apply sunscreen." Instead, there is ample record of people not only embracing the sun but actually worshiping it!

So how did we end up where we are today—thinking that the sun is something to be feared?

Dr. Michael Holick, professor of medicine, physiology, and biophysics at Boston University Medical Center, pulls the curtain back on a medical deception that I think is downright criminal. In his book *The Vitamin D Solution* he writes, "The simple answer lies in the fact that there are many billions of dollars to be made in emphasizing the only major medical downside of sun exposure (non-melanoma skin cancer) and not much money to be made in promoting the sun's many benefits. . . . The major culprits are the cosmetic wing of the pharmaceutical industry and what I consider to be some unenlightened dermatologists."

Wow! He goes on to say that the anti-sun lobby is so desperate to convince you of the sun's dangers and the need to buy their products that "its representatives will tell you with a straight face that if it's February in Boston and you're planning to walk to the corner store to buy a quart of milk or sit outside on your lunch break, you should wear sunscreen."

Jerry

Jerry lives as many of us live, in an *indoor* world. He sleeps in a house, drives to town in a tightly sealed automobile, works in a building, grabs a bite to eat at a nearby restaurant, and spends his free time watching television or hunched over the hobby table in his den. His time outdoors is brief and purposeful. Little did he know that his "shaded" life was affecting his health and causing many of the symptoms—chest pains, lack of sound sleep, muscle weakness, hypertension, the beginning stages of osteoporosis—that he presented to me on his first visit.

Jerry, like so many of us, is missing a vital element in God's Health Plan. The sun shining down on us wasn't put there so we could find our way to Wal-Mart without a flashlight. The sun is a foundational factor in gaining and maintaining optimum health—including the health of our hearts. We were made to be outside in the sunlight.

Remember how you felt the last time you spent a day outside with that "dangerous" sun lighting your play or your way? If you simply did what was necessary to keep from getting too much exposure and causing your skin to burn, you felt great, refreshed, invigorated. There's a reason for that.

Receiving adequate sunshine was not a problem for our ancestors. They worked outside, played outside, rode in open carriages or on horseback, and even socialized in outdoor venues such as parks, lakes, or rivers. What part of God's plan were they accepting into their lives—a part from which many of us fail to benefit? Two words: vitamin D.

I'd like to start a new ad campaign, which announces to the

world—in no uncertain terms—that sunlight is good for us. My motto would be "Got Sun?" I want to tell people that sunlight is a biblical prescription carrying a whole lot of science behind it.

Chemical Reactions Triggered by Sunlight

Vitamin D, which is actually a hormone, is needed for many important chemical reactions in the body. A few hours of sunshine each week usually do the trick. Many foods contain, or are fortified with, this important vitamin. There is a wide variety of supplements available for those who live a more "shaded" life. Vitamin D is stored and activated for use in the kidneys, but we must have enough stored in our bodies if our chemistry is going to function smoothly.

This hormone helps keep our cells from becoming diseased. In areas that receive little sunlight—near the North or South poles—there is a higher incidence of type 1 diabetes, rheumatoid arthritis, depression and suicide, multiple sclerosis, osteoporosis, and certain types of cancer. The bottom line is that we *must* have enough vitamin D in our bodies. The fact that each of us has an elaborate internal mechanism to regulate this hormone tells me, by simple logic, how important it is. Why would the liver, kidney, and parathyroid gland be involved if the Creator didn't have special plans for this particular vitamin?

Outdoor Deficiency

In this world of indoor living—especially for the elderly and those who call the far northern or southern latitudes home— vitamin D can be deficient. In this case, supplementation is essential. Most health professionals recommend 2,000 international units (IU) per day.

Scientists also tell us that too much calcium and animal protein can lower the amount of activated vitamin D in our systems. We are told that cow's milk is good for you, and it is—if you happen to be a calf. What we don't hear on television is that milk and animal proteins can adversely affect activated vitamin D and its reactions in the body.

Then there is another issue: our brains. Serotonin is an important brain messenger, or neurotransmitter. Low serotonin levels have been associated with many conditions, including depression and anxiety. Simply put, low levels of this transmitter put stress on our bodies. This is a worldwide problem and includes approximately nineteen million Americans who suffer from depression. The same number of Americans report experiencing chronic anxiety, with low levels of serotonin playing a role.

Here's the connection. Sun exposure generates a natural high by stimulating the release of "feel good" substances such as serotonin, dopamine, and beta-endorphins in our bodies. All three are dependent on vitamin D to function optimally. If we don't get enough sunlight, vitamin D levels are lower, thus decreasing the levels of serotonin. One treatment for depression and anxiety is sunlight. Another is to avoid animal protein.

"So," Jerry said, when I finished explaining this to him, "what's the bottom line, Doc?"

"Well," I said, "God created the sun for many reasons, one of which is to give us vitamin D. So here's what you do. Get outside for at least fifteen to thirty minutes, three or four days a week. If you ever move to a northern latitude, you might want to supplement with 2,000 IU of vitamin D each day. And keep in mind that adequate vitamin D protection requires exposure to sunlight for only one-fourth of the time required to burn the skin.

"Use common sense," I added. "Modest tanning is protective, sort of like putting sunglasses on your skin. Just don't overdo." Then I added with a smile, "And don't *underdo* either, okay?"

Jerry left my office, not with a prescription that needed to be filled at the local drugstore, but with one that can be satisfied with a walk around the neighborhood on a sunny day or an inexpensive supplement.

As I was writing this chapter, I couldn't help but think, *How many other chemical reactions are going awry of which we are not even aware—or ever will be aware—simply because we are not following the principles established by our Master Designer?* Why should I turn my back on His instructions when, by all accounts, they have to be irrefutably correct? In the first chapter of the first book of His Holy Word, I find His Health Plan in a complete and ready-to-use form. God knows how many hairs are on my head. Wouldn't He also know how to take care of not only my hairy head but also every other part of my body?

The world and its profit-seeking institutions want the subject of health to be difficult so that you and I will pay them big bucks to try to make us well. God's prescriptions for most chronic illnesses are free to everyone and are available everywhere. In my opinion, that's the best deal under the sun.

Moonlighting

There was another light that made its appearance on day four of Creation week (see Genesis 1:14). The moon, hanging silently over the land, became the official guardian of night, softly reflecting the sun's rays down onto the newly created plains and lofty mountains.

As far as I can tell, there is no medicinal power generated by moonlight unless you call romance medicinal. But it's what the moon represents that should be of extreme interest to us. On that fourth day, God created the day-night cycle—a light-dark system that repeats itself every twenty-four hours. Suddenly, our world had rhythm, as if some unseen clock in the universe had begun, marking hours of daylight followed by hours of nighttime. For some reason, the Creator knew that you and I would need this rhythm in our lives. Today, we know why. We have even given it a name—*circadian* rhythm.

In our modern world, we always seem to be on the go. There are more and more demands on our time. There are always meetings to attend, piles of paper in our in-boxes, busy social schedules to maintain, and responsibilities at home. I have even seen vacationers checking in with the office by cell phone as they attempt to jam beach umbrellas, coolers, and kids into the family Volvo. We cram more and more into each twenty-four-hour period, even trying to extend the period of daylight by an hour twice each year and changing how we mark time. The moon, hovering patiently overhead, is frequently ignored, lost in the blaze of streetlights, indoor illumination, and the steady glow of television and computer screens.

In the early part of the nineteenth century, Americans enjoyed about nine hours of sleep each night. Today, the average is down to seven hours—or less. And exactly what type of sleep are we getting? Every night we allow ourselves to get overstimulated by watching increasingly violent and often downright gross television programs, eating large meals, consuming caffeine-laced drinks and other stimulants, or staying on the job until exhaustion drives us home. This is not only occurring in America but is also becoming a worldwide trend.

What happened to God's rhythm? What happened to that day-night cycle that God gave us for a reason? Just think for a moment: we were designed to work taking care of the earth when the sun was up and to go to bed when the sun went down. But we are ignoring that design, bypassing it, totally rejecting the notion that such a rhythm exists. And we are doing so at our own peril.

As a cardiologist, I know that rest is definitely a treatment for cardiovascular disease. In the "old days" we frequently demanded bed rest after a heart attack. We need to rest in order to restore worn-out cells—and when I say rest, I mean *sleep*. We need a break from the constant sensory input that bombards. During true rest—the type that takes place in a darkened room with our eyes closed and the covers tucked comfortably under our chins, our stress hormones, which include epinephrine and cortisol, diminish.

While we sleep, increased activity of special white blood cells called "natural killer" cells, enhances our immune system and its ability to fight foreign substances like viruses, bacteria, and even some cancer cells. Our level of cortisol, associated with many diseases, also drops.

Adequate sleep helps build and maintain the neurotransmitters of the brain. Have you ever been sleep deprived and noticed how hard it is to think? Within our brains are special chemicals that enable it to communicate with every cell of our bodies. The disruption of these chemicals may result in depression and anxiety. Sleep also triggers the secretion of a growth hormone—another chemical important to our well-being.

My point is that adequate sleep assists *all* the functions of the body. When lack of rest alters the balance, a whole cascade of events may follow. If one chemical goes up, another chemical might go down, and the results can be anything but pleasant.

Getting Back into Rhythm

Isn't it time to get back into the rhythm God created on the fourth day? Isn't it time to stop fighting a rather obvious natural law that includes the sun and the moon as reminders of that law's presence in our lives?

Or we could just take pills. The drug industry hopes you'll make this choice. They'll be happy to sell you stimulants and relaxants to get you through your days and nights. They will be more than happy to set you up with stomach pills that mask the fact that the meal you ate late in the evening is still there in the morning when you "wake up." They will be happy to provide sleeping pills and tell you about "a good night's rest" when it was nothing more than a drug-induced stupor devoid of the benefits of true sleep. They will also not refuse to take your money as you battle the many illnesses that lack of sleep brings to the body. They probably have just the thing to address all those side effects from the stimulants and relaxants they sold you. No, they are not breaking any law by making these drugs available to you. It's you who may be a lawbreaker if you are turning your back on one of God's natural laws of health—sleep. But now you know better. Now *you're* in charge of your health.

In the treatment of all disease, rest and sleep are crucial. Ask yourself, *Do I get better gas mileage when I drive my car at fifty mph or at eighty mph? If I owned a champion racehorse, would I run that animal race after race without allowing it to rest between events? Am I not more important to my family, friends, and coworkers than a car or a horse?*

Don't be deceived into living a life devoid of good rest and sound sleep. Don't think that just because you can, you should. God placed the sun and the moon in the heavens as a reminder that although activity and work are essential to good health, so are rest and sleep. When you see that big round moon hovering over-head, do what you were designed to do. Turn off the TV and the computer, put the phone on silent, and turn out the lights. Let the moon guard your rest as your body takes advantage of that vital downtime to heal, rebuild, and prepare you for the day ahead.

Sleep tight!

11

DAY 5—A NEW SONG TO SING

THEN GOD SAID, "LET THE WATERS SWARM WITH FISH
AND OTHER LIFE. LET THE SKIES BE FILLED WITH BIRDS
OF EVERY KIND." SO GOD CREATED GREAT SEA CREATURES
AND EVERY LIVING THING THAT SCURRIES AND SWARMS IN
THE WATER, AND EVERY SORT OF BIRD—EACH PRODUCING
OFFSPRING OF THE SAME KIND. AND GOD SAW THAT IT WAS
GOOD. THEN GOD BLESSED THEM, SAYING, "BE FRUITFUL
AND MULTIPLY. LET THE FISH FILL THE SEAS, AND LET
THE BIRDS MULTIPLY ON THE EARTH."
AND EVENING PASSED AND MORNING CAME,
MARKING THE FIFTH DAY.

—GENESIS 1:20-23

I FIND SEVERAL INTERESTING things in the biblical account of day
five of Creation week—and they all pertain to our health.

First, I am so thankful that God did what He did on that day.
Can you imagine a walk in a forest devoid of birds? Think
about it. You hear the wind in the trees and the soft crunch of
your shoes on the leafy floor. But that's all. No laughing crows,
no chirping chickadees, no trilling wood thrushes, no hoot-
ing owls. That walk in the woods would be like listening to a
symphony played only by kettledrums, with the occasional wood
block thrown in.

The second interesting element of the account is found in these words: "God blessed them, saying, 'Be fruitful and multiply.'" Okay. God was talking to fish and birds. How do we know this? There was no one else to hear. Adam and Eve wouldn't show up until the next day. Nature hears the voice of God.

So here we have the Creator God making it clear to the birds of the air and the fish of the sea just what they are supposed to do now that they are here. They are supposed to make more birds and more fish.

When you look at the beginning words of God's statement to the fish and birds, you may notice something else. God "blessed" them.

In biblical language, a blessing is a conferring of purpose. Fathers blessed their sons, priests blessed their congregations, and prophets blessed entire nations. In each instance, it was made clear that through the blessing, the recipients were given a special responsibility, goal, or position in society.

I find it hard to believe that when God held His little seashore conference with the fish of the sea and the birds of the air, He was telling them that their main purpose in life was to be food. Death and the consumption of animals came later, after sin had infected the world. In Eden, birds and fish were to be on equal standing with all living creatures. They were blessed. They had purpose.

Making Music

Since I don't live underwater, I can't speak to the full benefit that aquatic creatures can bring to our lives, although they sure do a terrific job of keeping our oceans in good repair. A body of water devoid of fish is called "dead" for a reason. Not much of anything else grows there.

But I can talk about the impact birds have on people's

health—especially their hearts. That impact has to do with music.

Much of what we know about how to make melodies and harmonies we learned from the birds. They taught us phrasing, intonation, and breath control. More than one great master of music has left a forest with a tune echoing in his or her head that would later become a soul-stirring symphony. And when we hear played or sung notes moving among the scales with other notes supporting them, something amazing happens inside us.

It has been known for centuries that music can have a healing effect. David alluded to this in the psalms when he spoke of singing a new song (see Psalm 149). He took his cue from the birds and then added trumpets, flutes, stringed instruments, and his own voice (see Psalm 150). Whenever David was down, he knew a song of praise would lift him right back up. In fact, when King Saul was troubled, he would send for David to play and sing to him.

All living creatures brought into existence during Creation week were designed to sing praises. That bird sitting outside your window on a spring morning is delivering a tune God placed in its mind. Even whales sing. That whale drifting among the shadows of the deep is calling out in a song created by God Himself. When the angels announced Christ's birth, they didn't go around mumbling under their breath or writing out paper invitations. They praised God as a multitude, and the message was loud and clear! It filled the countryside and moved the hearts of simple shepherds.

Music can calm away the stresses of life. When a baby needs to go to sleep, we sing a lullaby. When we are worried or concerned, many of us hum softly to ourselves. The next time you watch a television program with a scene centered on true love and gentle compassion, listen to the supporting music. It's soft, rich, and soothing. Music is a powerful force for healing.

Medical Treatment

I was listening to the Wedgwood Trio and praying for the right words to place in this chapter about music as a medical treatment. The Wedgwood Trio is made up of three musicians who have been playing and singing together since the 1960s. One plays an upright bass, the second strums a guitar, and the third rotates among several instruments, including a harmonica.

They have always performed songs filled with praise and hope. As I listened to their beautiful melodies and harmonies, I found myself beginning to relax. My heart rate and breathing slowed. A peace came over me. I believe the Holy Spirit filled my mind with thoughts and scenes I needed to include in this chapter. I found that, just like the birds of Eden, music offered a special way of preparing to commune with the One who made me, a special aspect of worship.

I'm not naive enough to think that the music I enjoy is the only music God uses to touch hearts. Making or hearing music is very individualized. Sometimes, if it suits God's purpose, there may be no instrument or voice involved at all. Some find healing in the whisper of the wind as it moves through the trees. For others, it might be the ocean's roar that brings peace to their souls. It could be chirping birds or buzzing insects that lower the blood pressure and slow the hearts of still others. That is why all nature sings some type of song. God's creations sing for a reason. They, as we, were designed to praise God through their songs. If you are like me, your favorite type of "music" might include the absolute stillness at the end of a hectic day. Take a moment and listen. What do you hear?

The Source of the Song

When it comes to music, what really matters is the heart of the musician. What matters is the source of the song.

Like everything else God created, sin has reshaped and mutated the music of this world. The wrong type of music can actually damage our chemistry, causing our bodies to respond in unhealthy ways. Some very heinous crimes have been committed while loud, dissonant music was blaring from nearby boom boxes or on the family stereo. There's a reason why many soldiers go into battle with loud, strident tunes playing in their earbuds.

Dissonant tunes, boom boxes, and heinous crimes didn't exist in Eden when God called the birds into being. The song He gave them to sing—the song with which He blessed them—was simple and beautiful. It was a melody that continually filled their hearts with joy and praise.

We were made to praise God in song, and when we do, we are following the owner's manual, even if we don't understand the exact physiology. Music can be more powerful than any pill.

When was the last time you felt poorly after singing a song of praise to God? I'll bet never, because that is not going to happen. There's a chemical reaction behind that good feeling. When we are happy, our endorphin levels increase. The stress chemicals diminish. When David needed a lift, he sang. When the birds wanted to respond to God's love on that fifth day of Creation, they sang.

The music is in you. The blessing has already been given. The healing is waiting to happen. Sing!

12

DAY 6—SOMEONE TO LOVE

THEN GOD SAID, "LET THE EARTH PRODUCE EVERY
SORT OF ANIMAL, EACH PRODUCING OFFSPRING OF
THE SAME KIND—LIVESTOCK, SMALL ANIMALS THAT
SCURRY ALONG THE GROUND, AND WILD ANIMALS."
AND THAT IS WHAT HAPPENED. . . .
THEN GOD SAID, "LET US MAKE HUMAN BEINGS IN OUR
IMAGE, TO BE LIKE US. THEY WILL REIGN OVER THE FISH
IN THE SEA, THE BIRDS IN THE SKY, THE LIVESTOCK,
ALL THE WILD ANIMALS ON THE EARTH, AND THE SMALL
ANIMALS THAT SCURRY ALONG THE GROUND."
SO GOD CREATED HUMAN BEINGS IN HIS OWN IMAGE. . . .
AND EVENING PASSED AND MORNING CAME,
MARKING THE SIXTH DAY.

—GENESIS 1:24, 26-27, 31

AS I ENTERED THE ROOM, my hand was barely off the doorknob
when David exclaimed, "Doctor Marcum, I know exactly why
day six is in God's Health Plan! I figured it out all by myself
just by reading the Bible and praying. I didn't need *Wikipedia*,
a library, or a theologian. You are right. The Bible *can* be 'figured
out' by a guy like me."

Inwardly, I knew David would need me less and less now.
God was talking directly to his heart.

The sixth day of Creation was a busy one by any standard.

Imagine the work that would go into creating—from scratch, mind you—an elephant. Where do you put everything? Or how about a cat? Or a zebra? Think of the creative power necessary to form a single living ant. Amazing!

Then there are human beings. These creatures would enjoy the added benefit of being able to be innovative and generate technology to help people live better lives, to build skyscrapers, airplanes, and cell phones. Humans would be able to think and reason in ways the animals could not. And—this is important to remember—men and women were created in the image of God Himself. They were unique, special, highly intelligent, and for all intents and purposes, godlike.

After Adam was created, God made it very clear what He had in mind as far as man's relationship with animals is concerned. "The LORD God . . . brought [the animals] to the man to see what he would call them, and the man chose a name for each one. He gave names to all the livestock, all the birds of the sky, and all the wild animals" (Genesis 2:19-20).

Let me ask you a question. What happens when you name a stray dog or cat that shows up at your doorstep? That's right—it becomes something special to you. In your mind, it now belongs to you. It's part of your world. In other words, you begin to love it.

That is what God could have had in mind when He asked Adam to name every living creature on earth. God wanted Adam to experience that sense of ownership, responsibility, and love so that when he governed the animal kingdom, every decision he made concerning God's creatures would flow from a heart filled with respect and a deep commitment to each animal's safety and comfort. That is not exactly the image that comes to mind when you think of the thousands of slaughterhouses sprinkled about our globe. Not exactly the image one gets when sitting down to devour a meal with cooked meat at its center. God's Health

Plan took into consideration the well-being of both humans *and animals.*

Healing Pets

The health benefits for people who interact in a loving, support-ive way with animals are well documented. One study suggests that spending a little time with the family pet may relieve greater amounts of stress than taking a pill, talking with a best friend, or even conversing with one's spouse.

Sometimes, it seems, animals can even work miracles. Consider this from a recent ABC News report. A golden retriever called Janie walked down the hall of the Cedars-Sinai Medical Center in Los Angeles and breezed into the room of a patient who had refused to talk with anyone in weeks. Then Janie did something that the best medical treatments had been unable to do. As she put her paws on the edge of the bed, the formerly uncommunicative patient leaned over, began stroking Janie's ears, and started talking.

Researchers across the country are discovering that pets can do everything from reducing blood pressure during times of intense stress to easing the pain of loneliness.

Animals are even therapeutic for people with Alzheimer's, says Dr. John W. Tracy, a family practice physician in Fancy Gap, Virginia, because they get people to look inside themselves a little bit.

In a study at Purdue University, researchers examined the effect of the presence of a fish tank on patients with Alzheimer's. Before the fish tank, many patients at a particular nursing home often got up and wandered away from the table during meals, which reduced the amount of nutrition they received. But after the staff installed an aquarium in the dining room and stocked it with colorful fish, patients remained in their seats and ate their entire meals in peace.

Sarah

Sarah had been my patient for four years. I was treating her for atrial fibrillation—a condition in which the upper chamber of the heart beats rapidly. She had done well with the treatment, and we both were encouraged.

During those four years I had also gotten to know Sarah's husband, Mac. Mac loved two things: driving his truck and caring for Sarah. They always came to the office together and were obviously very much in love.

Then Mac became sick with pneumonia and died suddenly at the age of eighty-two. When Sarah came back to visit a month after the funeral, she seemed totally and understandably lost. She was a woman of faith and turned to God for help, but naturally she still carried a broken heart. Her blood pressure was up, she was not sleeping well at night, and her memory was beginning to slip. Her family was being supportive, but without Mac, the love of Sarah's life, her health was fading.

I had seen this before. When a loved one passes away, the stress from the loss places an extreme burden on a body. If something is not done quickly, damage can result. Yes, people can die of broken hearts.

One of my patients had an extra dog, and I suggested to Sarah that she adopt this lovable ball of fur. Three months passed, and when Sarah came in for her quarterly checkup, she was a completely different woman. Sarah told me about her new Maltese, and though she still missed Mac, she had learned to love that dog, and the pooch had responded with an overflow of love in return. I wasn't surprised. Animals—as designed by God—can help our chemistry by giving us unconditional love.

I experience this with my own dogs, Max and Daphne. My wife really does not care for them when they insist on doing their business in the house, but whenever I come home from work, they are always there to greet me—making me feel as if I'm the most important human in the world. When I must stay up late at night, they patiently sit at my feet. Max and Daphne lower my stress levels by showing me love.

Animals enrich our lives—amaze us, cheer us up, calm us down, allay our fears, and bring our world to life. That was the Creator's intent when He made them for us to enjoy. A large part of God's Health Plan includes friendly, loving interaction with *all* the creatures of this world. In fact, we are all healers when we make others laugh, help them feel good about themselves, or show them love. We change their chemistry for the good. Animals are prescriptions for the world, and we can be the same.

But God had one more healthy surprise waiting for Adam on that sixth day—Eve!

Here's an interesting fact: married people tend to live longer and healthier lives than single people. Actually, perhaps I'd better restate that with one word added. *Happily* married people tend to live longer and healthier lives than their single friends. Scientists conclude that it probably has to do with the lowering of stress that comes when people's hearts are filled with love, when the focus is on someone other than themselves, and when they have someone with whom to share life's ups and downs. Whatever the reason, God created the institution of marriage for our health. It's part of His plan.

And where there's marriage, more than likely there is family.

Matthew

Matthew had been in the intensive care unit for a week when I got to know him. He was fifty-four and suffered from an infection on his leg—a condition that had started on a camping trip the month before. Matthew hadn't paid much attention to it at first.

But this infection did not clear up. One of the conditions that made Matthew more susceptible was the fact that he was a diabetic, and diabetes inhibits the immune system. The infection moved from the leg into the bloodstream, and Matthew became very sick, with high temperatures and low blood pressure. The infection also damaged the mitral valve in his heart and caused a dangerous leak. Because fluid was building up in his lungs, Matthew was put on a ventilator, and surgery to replace the leaky valve was scheduled as soon as possible. We all feared he would die. The numbers did not look good. Even though we had done everything we could, we honestly did not know whether he'd pull through.

One thing I did notice about Matthew was that he had a very strong family. The kids, his wife, his in-laws, and his mom and dad were all there supporting him, praying for him, helping in any way possible, and showing their love and concern.

I believe there is power in family because the original social unit on this earth—the original human structure that God set up in Eden—was the family. Adam had Eve. Eve had Adam. In time, there would be little Adams and Eves running around, filling their lives with happy laughter. Love would spread from person to person. But that was just the beginning.

The family was also designed to be the place to worship and learn about God, to help people survive and make a living, to belong, and after sin entered the world, to provide a safe harbor in which to weather the storms of life.

Matthew enjoyed this type of environment in his own family, and I believe this aided his healing. No, I can't measure its benefit on paper or chart the results on a graph, but the effect of his family's support was real, and my patient's ability to come through such a stressful ordeal is proof that in so many cases, family makes a healing difference.

Unfortunately, the world tells us, "Family isn't all that important. Kids don't need a mom *and* a dad. Hey, you can have it all—a career, a big home, and a loving family." But while people live in light of this lie, the divorce rate is rising. Families are dissolving right before our eyes, and society and individuals are suffering untold misery because of it.

In this fast-paced world, we are forgetting the healing power of family. This is where love is learned, where God is revealed, where worship is expressed. When Christ came to this earth, He spent more time in a family unit than He did in active ministry. During this family time, He was learning and growing. When His ministry work finally did begin, He had the tools and support network necessary to keep Him going in the face of agonizing barriers. How many young people can say the same thing about their family structure today?

I'll bet you never thought of family as a treatment for disease. Well, it is. A good family will change our chemistry. When this precious, healing unit is torn apart, we have a much harder time learning about love the way God intended it to be. More and more families are being torn apart contrary to the original plan. Children from divorced homes have a harder time trusting God, because they get their sense of who God is from their experience with their earthly fathers. Moms are working outside the home to provide for the family and then come home to care for the house and put meals on the table. They have less time and energy to devote to parenting. When family is minimized, stress increases, and everyone gets shortchanged. Family is a healing force. Just ask Matthew.

One More Thing

So here we are, six days into Creation week. Adam and Eve are standing hand in hand, surveying all that God has done and reveling in the beauty and majesty of every tree, flower, and animal. They are breathing deeply of the nature-scented air, drinking from pure, sparkling streams, eating of the fresh fruits and vegetables growing in abundance all about them. What more could they possibly need?

That is when God spoke again. We don't know what words He used, but His meaning was clear because we read that "the Lord God took the man and put him in the Garden of Eden to work it and take care of it" (Genesis 2:15, NIV).

Work? Did God just instruct Adam and Eve to *work*? Why? They had everything they needed: a beautiful Garden home, food, fellowship with each other, and the animals! Why work?

Because God knew that physical activity—especially physical activity resulting in a feeling of accomplishment or satisfaction—is good for our health. Activity is also good for our brains. Mentally active people tend to enjoy an increased clarity of thought well into old age. Spiritually active folk who attend church regularly, volunteer, and get involved in meeting the needs of others tend to remain closer to God as the years roll by.

God created us with legs instead of roots for a reason. We were designed to move and be active while taking care of the earth. Over the course of centuries, especially the last fifty years, we have been moving less and less. Such inactivity is taking a tremendous chemical toll on our bodies.

Chemical toll? That's right. Activity enables our bodies to make chemicals that help lower our blood pressure, strengthen our immune system, and make our bones stronger. It helps us burn fat—a growing concern in this country where obesity rates are skyrocketing. As a matter of fact, fat has its own scientific name now—the *endocannabinoid* system. This system is capable of making chemicals of its own—chemicals that damage the body. It's as if all the fat we are carrying around has a life of its own! Activity, exercise, movement—whatever you want to call it—helps keep us away from having that endocannabinoid system stress our other systems.

Sam

Sam ventured into my office a few years ago. He easily weighed in at four hundred pounds, but he stood only about five-and-a-half feet tall. I knew right away that his endocannabinoid system (i.e., body fat) was changing him chemically. His blood sugar was high. He had elevated blood pressure and suffered from diabetes.

The burden of carrying around the extra weight was causing painful wear on his joints. Because of all the prescription medications he was on, he was suffering from numerous side effects—impotence being one of them. In short, Sam felt lousy.

He was not alone. Up to 60 percent of Americans are over-weight, and the industrialized world is "growing" at similar rates.

I explained to Sam that too many calories and too little exercise over a period of time were his true enemies. Excess fat was causing his body to work harder. This raised blood pressure, increased the workload on his heart, elevated cholesterol levels, and multiplied his chances of developing diabetes. Fat causes the body to handle sugar incorrectly, creating extra insulin, and that is not a good thing either.

"What do you mean?" he asked.

"Well," I continued, "insulin is a substance that helps sugar move into the body's cells. High levels of blood sugar may also cause the blood pressure to increase. The increased amount of fat causes the liver to handle fats abnormally, turning fat into artery-clogging cholesterol. And not only does the risk of cardiovascular disease increase, but the risk of cancer and asthma skyrockets as well. In fact, women who gain more than twenty pounds after the age of eighteen double the risk of postmenopausal breast cancer. Every two pounds of extra weight increases the risk of arthritis by at least 9 percent. Bottom line, Sam? All the diseases from which you are suffering are really symptoms resulting from being overweight. If you lose the weight, you lose the symptoms."

Sam's mouth dropped open. "No one has ever put it to me like that," he said. "Do you think a weight-loss pill would help?"

I explained to Sam that we are being deceived by the many diets and weight-loss plans out there. These can be not only expensive but dangerous. "There are no quick fixes," I told him. "As a matter of fact, some diet pills have caused major health issues. Many of the diets and exercise plans just leave a person unhappy and stressed out. A person spends a lot of money, loses a bit of weight, then quickly gains it back again. And another cycle starts."

I could not help but feel the pain and frustration my patient was feeling. Sam, like many of us, wanted a quick fix. He wanted more medication to help with his symptoms. But I knew that unless something really changed, he would be back in my office within months—possibly with even more health problems. "If you really want to feel better," I told him, "you're going to have to start living better. It's a journey, not a destination. Are you serious about this? Because I sure am."

Sam nodded. "Just tell me what I have to do, Dr. Marcum."

Together, we worked out a plan—a health plan for Sam.

He could barely walk across the room when we started. So we set small but important goals. At first he walked one minute a couple of times a day. That's right. One minute. Then we began to increase his walk time to five minutes, then ten, then twenty. In a matter of weeks, he began to feel better, and we took him off a blood pressure medication.

Next, Sam's walk spanned thirty minutes, then forty minutes a day. He started to feel even better, and the dose on his diabetes medications was lowered.

He began to walk faster and added some light strength training. His chemistry responded in some amazing ways as he experienced undeniable proof that people were designed to be active.

Other changes occurred as well. Now, after four years, Sam does forty-five minutes of aerobic exercises with twenty minutes of strength training six days a week. Then he takes one day a week off to rest. He has lost two hundred pounds, no longer has high blood pressure, is not diabetic, suffers fewer joint pains, is not depressed, and doesn't stagger under the debilitating side effects of medications. In fact, he now takes one medication— for his seasonal allergies.

Today, how many doctors include on their prescription tablets the word *walk*? How many sit down with their patients and outline a workable walking program? Some do. But most, I'm afraid, would say, "Who has time for that?"

"Give 'em a pill and send 'em a bill." That's the motto of so many medical professionals in this modern, overweight society. But God knew exactly what we needed. The antidote for so many of the diseases from which we suffer today was staring Adam and Eve squarely in the face. "Here's your garden," the Creator told them. "Tend it. Care for it. Keep moving. Keep working. Be active!"

We may not be tending gardens these days, but the principle remains. We were not meant to sit and stare at something. We were made to move. It's part of the plan.

The Bridge

I recall a story told to me by a crew member who worked for a Christian television ministry. The production team was in San

Francisco filming a documentary on the subject of suicide. Now don't get me wrong. The crew wasn't there because the hard-working folk who live in San Francisco are suicide prone. It's *what's* in San Francisco that drew the filmmakers to that part of California.

Stretching majestically over the inlet leading to that beautiful bay is the Golden Gate Bridge, a marvel of engineering and, apparently, a powerful magnet for people who want to end their lives.

While the crew was setting up their equipment in order to interview one of the security guards at the entrance to the bridge, the scanner in the guard booth rattled to life. "Attention all security personnel. We've got a jumper midspan. I repeat. We've got a jumper midspan." Sure enough, while the production team was getting ready to talk with a guard about the many suicides that had taken place on the bridge, a small, foreign-built car had stopped in the middle of the center span. The driver, a young man wearing worn jeans and a T-shirt, had unhurriedly exited the vehicle, walked to the railing, climbed to the upper pole, hesitated for just a moment, and then stepped out into space. His life ended with a silent splash far below.

In his car he had left a note with these words carefully written across its wrinkled surface: "Happiness is someone to love, something to do, and something to look forward to."

On the sixth day of Creation, God provided all three of these requirements for happiness for Adam and Eve. He gave them someone to love. He showed them a garden waiting to be tended and a world filled with animals eager for attention and care so Adam and Eve would always have something to do. And, finally, He told them, "Be fruitful and multiply. Fill the earth and govern it" (Genesis 1:28). Earth's first couple could look forward to becoming earth's first parents—sharing the same flawless creative power that had formed them in the first place.

Biblical scholars will tell you that on the sixth day of Creation week, God made animals and human beings. This is true. But He also set in place the most powerful healing agent this world would ever see. On day six, God created love between people.

13

DAY 7—HEALING REST

ON THE SEVENTH DAY GOD HAD FINISHED HIS WORK OF
CREATION, SO HE RESTED FROM ALL HIS WORK. AND GOD
BLESSED THE SEVENTH DAY AND DECLARED IT HOLY,
BECAUSE IT WAS THE DAY WHEN HE RESTED
FROM ALL HIS WORK OF CREATION.

—GENESIS 2:2-3

AT THE END of a long day's work, American cowboys liked nothing better than to kick off their boots and sit by a crackling fire, eager to savor the coming night's rest. On the seventh day of Creation week, God invited us to do the same. It's part of His amazing Health Plan.

The word *rest* in Genesis 2:2 also means "to cease" or "to stop doing what one has been doing." So, in essence, on the seventh day, God stopped the creative work he had been doing. Today, Christians know that day as the "Sabbath," or "day of rest."

Generations after Creation, from the summit of Mount

Sinai, God reminded the children of Israel just how He wanted the holy day observed. Listen to His words as recorded in Exodus 20, starting with verse 8. "Remember to observe the Sabbath day by keeping it holy. You have six days each week for your ordinary work, but the seventh day is a Sabbath day of rest dedicated to the LORD your God. On that day no one in your household may do any work. . . . For in six days the LORD made the heavens, the earth, the sea, and everything in them; but on the seventh day he rested. That is why the LORD blessed the Sabbath day and set it apart as holy" (Exodus 20:8-11).

I don't know how you feel about this, but it seems to me God is demonstrating a genuine concern about how we spend our Sabbath hours—how we "keep" the Sabbath. By using the word "remember," He indicates this was part of the original Health Plan, which could easily be forgotten. Resting is not often equated with a change in the body's chemistry or even with a treatment for ailments. But resting is required for the maintenance of the entire system. As I tell my patients, we get better gas mileage when we drive at fifty rather than at eighty miles an hour. At the end of Creation week, God was concerned for our future health.

Today, scientists are discovering an interesting fact. Rest— or ceasing from our labors—is not only good for our minds but also good for our bodies.

In our fast-paced, exhausting lives, insomnia is running rampant. People are gulping down millions of sedatives and tranquilizers, desperate for the rest that can restore their energy. Those who take no break from the daily grind suffer increased bouts of infections and are often depressed. They become irritable, lose their tempers more often, and can find even the simplest tasks overwhelming. When our minds and bodies do not get sufficient rest, burnout waits just around the corner.

Being sleep or rest deprived turns on the stress cascade we have mentioned, which is not a good thing over the long haul.

When God was creating this world, He was looking far beyond the needs of just Adam and Eve. Using His infinite and eternal mind of love, He was scanning the future of His creation, seeing you and me languishing in a world overtaken by sin. He saw our need to escape from the pain of life, from the hurt and sorrow He knew we would face in this broken world. So, on that last day of Creation week, He became a visual aid for us to study—a perfect template around which we could fashion our lives. On the seventh day, God rested. And so should we.

Sabbath rest means a lot more than Sabbath *sleep*. The Creator made the day holy (i.e., set apart for a special purpose) so we would have a day each week in which we could change our focus, slow our pace, and redirect our motivations. It is a day in which we can stop worrying about ourselves and spend time blessing others. How? Many find opportunities for Sabbath rest by attending church, listening to God speak to them through sermons, getting involved in outreach programs, singing in the choir, teaching in one of the children's classes, or greeting visitors at the door.

Others seek the solitude of nature, roaming forest paths or walking deserted beaches. Some spend the hours of the Sabbath reading or listening to inspiring music. There are many ways to rest on God's holy day. And, yes, if it's needed, some close their eyes and sleep, spending hours cradled by the knowledge that they are giving their bodies the much-needed opportunity to recharge.

Rest, in all its forms, allows the body to renew itself. It aids in the healing of injuries and infections—including emotional traumas. Rest strengthens the body's immune system, helping to protect against disease. And proper rest can actually add length to life. Is it any wonder, then, why God created the Sabbath? Why He included it in His powerful Health Plan?

Some people say I have an active imagination, and perhaps I do. But there's an image I like to form in my mind when I see the sun slipping below the horizon at the end of the sixth day of the week. I've spent the afternoon getting ready to enjoy the hours of the Sabbath, and as the Sabbath day begins, I imagine Jesus standing above the setting sun, arms outstretched, and looking right at me. From His lips I hear the words recorded in Matthew 11:28-29: "Come to me, all of you who are weary and carry heavy burdens, and I will give you rest. Take my yoke upon you. Let me teach you, because I am humble and gentle at heart, and you will find rest for your souls."

I invite you to partake of God's special rest—God's *Sabbath* rest. Although He loves to be worshiped any day of the week and eagerly looks forward to spending time with you, He specifically asked us to work six days and rest a day. He could have worked two and rested one or worked nine and rested one, but the Creator knew this was how He designed us to function optimally, work six days and rest. There is only one day He set aside as holy, only one day He included in His powerful Health Plan. That's the Sabbath—the one He created way back in Eden and designed specifically to nurture and protect our health and well-being.

As a behavioral cardiologist, I can say from experience that rest is definitely a treatment for cardiovascular disease. We need rest to restore our bodies and replace worn-out and dead cells. We need a break from the sensory input that constantly bombards us. During physical rest, our stress hormones diminish.

I believe not only in physical rest but also in a mental rest, during which we renew the spiritual component of our lives. Would God have given us a principle that was not beneficial for our long-term health?

Kaye

Kaye came to my office as winter was fading into the expectation
of spring. Although she was fifty-two, her olive skin showed few
wrinkles. Her intelligent green eyes shone with a hint of hope
as she began telling me the reason for her visit to the mountains
of eastern Tennessee, far from her home on the Eastern Shore
of Maryland. Five feet eight inches tall, she boasted an athletic
build. To look at her, one would never know she'd been ill for
many years.

Kaye carried a strong family history of heart disease. She had
experienced her first bypass surgery at forty-three and a repeat
performance at fifty. As I looked through her well-organized
records, I noticed she had already seen some of the most
respected cardiologists in the country. She was already receiving
every possible, scientifically proven treatment and was coming to
me, as many patients do, for a second opinion, to see if anything
else could be offered to improve her condition.

As we visited, I discovered a bit more about her. She had
smoked cigarettes throughout her twenties but had kicked that
habit completely. Now she operated a very successful business
that kept her traveling much of the time. Her two children
attended college, and her husband, an attorney, had an equally
demanding career. She admitted she rarely did anything "just
for Kaye."

My visitor was on all the right medications at the correct
dosages. Her blood pressure, cholesterol levels, and diet were
exemplary, and she exercised forty-five minutes a day. But she
still felt miserable much of the time.

Finally, to make sure all the bases were covered, I began to
explore how much time she spent in rest. I knew lack of rest is
a gigantic stressor that is often overlooked. She seemed puzzled
and a little surprised as I probed this aspect of her life. Sensing

her unspoken questions, I began to explain why I wanted to know about her rest patterns.

The Hidden Culprit

When God created the universe, He also designed certain laws that would govern its operation. Sir Isaac Newton was the first to clearly explain one such principle. It dictates that if you jump off a cliff, there will be severe consequences. This law remains in full force whether you believe in it or not. Gravity is well known to any child who has ever tried to fly.

I explained to Kaye that just as there are laws holding the universe together, there are certain laws governing how well our bodies function. One of those irrefutable, seldom recognized yet extremely powerful laws is the need for rest. Like gravity, we ignore it at our own peril.

I told my visitor that our bodies, when healthy, maintain a certain chemical profile—just enough of this, just enough of that. But the profile is not static. It changes to meet demands. If we get an infection, our bodies heat themselves up to kill the germs. When we sit in the sun too long, our bodies release moisture through perspiration to cool them off. When our minds sense danger, our bodies prepare to either face the foe or get out of Dodge—fast. Most of what happens in our bodies takes place as the result of changes in our chemistry, which in many cases is a good thing.

However, infections and creeping tigers aren't the only foes we face. Work-, environment-, or relationship-related stresses, chronic illnesses, malnutrition brought on by unhealthy food choices, lack of adequate water intake, sedentary lifestyles, even watching the six o'clock news can alter our chemistry in some rather profound ways. Our bodies, sensing the strain, try to meet the demand by making adjustments. In the case of illness, bodies do what they need to do to bring about healing, which may include shutting down or altering some important bodily functions. In other words, our bodies are trying to meet the challenge and then return to a more balanced state as quickly as possible.

But what if the challenge is never ending? What if the stress continues day after day, week after week, year after year? Then our bodies remain in an altered, unbalanced state, their chemistry profiles far from what they should be—like operating a car with its brakes on or trying to build a house without adequate tools or materials.

This brought our conversation back to the law of rest. Rest is an important factor in "resetting" the body, allowing it to return to a more balanced condition. Without an adequate and regular release from tensions or everyday challenges, our chemistry begins to change for the worse.

As I continued, I could tell I had sparked Kaye's interest. She was especially intrigued when I posed this rhetorical question: "Would you rather take a prescription medication to change your chemistry, or would you like to learn how to rest and accomplish the same thing and a whole lot more?"

I explained that the God of the universe worked six days when creating this earth. Then He rested on the seventh day. He could have worked one day and rested the next, or worked four days and then taken a break. But God chose to rest on the seventh day. He even went so far as to bless it (see Genesis 2:2-3), setting it aside for a special purpose. Apparently, our Creator understood that a ratio of one in seven—one day of rest for six days of honest labor—brought about just the right balance in the human body. That is why He created the law of rest right along with fresh air, pure water, palm trees, and aardvarks.

I then reemphasized that when we violate one of God's

laws—whether we believe the law exists or not—our chemistry is altered. After all, the Creator knows how His creation is supposed to operate. That is why He put His laws of health—the laws so many of us ignore or reject or don't even know about—into place. When we fail to rest, our chemistry changes for the worse. As a result, stress is placed on *all* the systems of the body.

The Cycles of Life

That weekly rest was only part of the picture. God also created the day-night cycles we call circadian rhythms. Every one of us operates under their steady cadence. The body is actually hardwired to slow down at night and speed up during the day—a cycle determined by two hormones, melatonin and serotonin.

In today's world, this natural rhythm is often broken. Think of the late-night eating that doesn't allow our gastrointestinal systems to rest. Stimuli such as television, the Internet, iPods, and cell phones continue to bombard our systems long after the sun goes down. Then, because of our lack of adequate sleep at night, we chemically stimulate our bodies to keep going the next day. Day after day, week after week, month after month, and year after year, the pattern continues. Sometimes we doze during the day—at times with tragic results. When this day-night cycle is compromised, our chemistry is altered.

I asked Kaye, "Have you ever been sleep deprived or worked a long time without rest?"

She nodded.

"Well," I continued, "under those conditions, the law of rest is being violated. The physical, emotional, and cognitive functions of the body are damaged. Stress is placed on the entire system."

During these times, our stress chemicals—including epinephrine and cortisol—rise. They, in turn, alter other chemical reactions in the body. If this condition goes on long enough, the body can be damaged by a heart attack, ulcers, poor digestion, tight muscles, high blood pressure, palpitations, headaches, strokes, weakened immune systems, and a host of other pains—all because we've ignored God's law of rest. Most chronic diseases that plague modern society contain stress as a major component.

True Confession

At this point, I asked Kaye rather bluntly, "Have you been violating God's natural law of rest? Are you jumping off a ten-story building?"

I watched my visitor as a new understanding dawned in her mind. It was obvious I had hit upon the one area of her life that she had allowed to become out of control. Gently I suggested that making some small but consistent changes to her life could greatly improve her chemistry. If additional and regular rest could be added to her treatment regimen, it just might penetrate to the very core of her problem. "After all," I said, "why would the God of the universe mention rest if it weren't important?

"Kaye," I continued, "don't you want the best for your children?"

"Of course," she responded emphatically, unsure of why I had asked such a question.

"Well," I said, "God wants the best for you, too."

After a short pause, she looked at me with genuine interest. "Dr. Marcum," she said, "I don't mean to put you on the spot, but I really want to know, how do *you* rest?"

I explained that I try to get adequate sleep at night, although call nights are challenging. I try to faithfully keep to the seven-day cycle God designed. On the seventh day of each week, I try to get more rest—physical and mental. I sleep longer and do my best to not think about my work. I spend time worshiping and listening to the God who created me. I plan special activities for my family, which might include going on a nature adventure, eating a special meal together, spending time with friends, helping someone in need, or giving an extra measure of love where needed—anything to break my everyday routine.

How people rest, I explained, is personal and depends on their definition of the word. For some, resting is climbing a mountain. For others, it might be snoozing in the shade of a backyard tree. Still others find rest in association with their church family or simply strolling through the park. The key is to learn how *God* wants you to rest and then stick to it, realizing it is vital to optimal health. Rest is necessary to prevent *and treat* every known disease.

Our session was coming to an end, and I once more explained that when we live in harmony with God's laws, our chemistry improves, stress is relieved, and healing occurs. What Kaye needed most was true rest—healing rest—a powerful and gracious gift from God.

I believe on that late winter day Kaye added a new treatment to her regimen, one without adverse side effects and filled with eternal benefits. She left my office with a fresh understanding and a desire to learn more about God's timeless laws for building and maintaining optimum health. Her healing had already begun.

Worship

My conversation with Kaye got me to thinking not only about Sabbath rest but also about Sabbath worship. As Christians, we tend to spend at least a portion of those holy hours engaged in some sort of worship. For many, the homage we pay is not to our Creator but to something very different—and that difference can take a toll on our health. Let me explain.

Kelli, my fourteen-going-on-twenty-year-old daughter, asked me why so many people make such a big deal about football and other sports. I must admit, we as a society, myself included, spend considerable time on sports of all sorts. I explained that the game is exciting, fun to play and watch, and that competition between equally matched teams allows each player's skills to be put to the test. That's about all I could say. While those of us who love the game see a combination of strategy and strength on the field, all Kelli sees are really big men running into one another and knocking one another down. To a fourteen-year-old girl, that must seem very strange indeed.

Football also teaches me something about God and about worship. We have been learning about biblical treatments to help change our chemistry. Our Creator God is constant. He does not change. The laws He set in motion during Creation week are also constant. It makes perfect sense that God, like the coach of a winning football team, would give us the best game plan to care for our bodies. It also makes perfect sense to me that Satan would target his tricks at that plan.

Which brings me back to Sabbath worship. While I certainly enjoy a good football game as much as the next guy, I know you and I were not designed to *worship* football—or any other sport for that matter. That is why it seems strange to me that in the fall, hundreds of thousands of us will flock to games each Saturday and Sunday. Not only that, but we also spend hours watching sports on TV, reading about our favorite teams and players in the newspaper, and listening to guys on the radio go on and on about the next game or the one just played. Even water-cooler conversations usually focus on sports. Baseball, basketball, NASCAR, golf, tennis, soccer—the list seems endless. Again, while there is absolutely nothing wrong with these sports per se, there is a problem when they become objects of worship. We were designed to worship our Creator, not some sports team or pumped-up jock.

Wouldn't it be great if our places of worship experienced such growing attendance, with hundreds of thousands of people paying money, standing in line for hours to pay homage to our Creator? Wouldn't it be great if people wore clothes proclaiming the greatness of God rather than the logo of a local sports team? What if talk shows on the radio and television were praising God and talking about how we could enhance our worship of Him? What if, in addition to a sports page, our local newspaper had a worship page? What if, at the watercooler, we spoke of God and His greatness in our lives, sharing with our coworkers ways to know Him better?

I can answer those "what if" questions. We would be healthier. We would live longer. We would have a lot less stress and disease in our lives. Why is that? Because we become like who and what we worship. Our chemistry improves when we shift our focus to the One who designed us. In other words, worship can be a powerful treatment if what we worship fills our hearts with joy and love.

Of course, the evil one wants to discredit the Creation Health Plan and those who proclaim the chemical importance of worshiping the true God. But we know better. Health has always been, and always will be, about what *and who* we worship.

"Come and See!"

I wish I could have been there on the first Sabbath in Eden. If you will allow me one more flight of imagination, I see Adam and Eve strolling through their sunlit garden, marveling at the animals—each of which has been named by Adam himself. They pause and drink deeply from a clear-flowing stream or pluck a brightly colored fruit from an overhanging limb.

They listen to the symphony echoing from the trees as birds fill the air with their song. The grass underfoot is soft and welcoming, and they settle down to nap as the whispering breezes carry them gently into slumber. They feel a deep and safe love for each other and for the world they inhabit.

Then they hear a voice calling, "Adam? Eve? Come with Me. There are many more beauties I want to show you."

I can hear their cries of joy as they run to the arms of the Creator Himself. Like children, they follow Him along verdant paths and beside glass-clear lakes, marveling at the amazing sights and sounds at each step, laughing and smiling as God reveals His detailed handiwork.

How is it possible for them to be so happy? Because God's Health Plan is in full force in their lives. There has been nothing damaging in their existence—nothing that can diminish their vitality. They are healthy in mind, body, and spirit. They are in perfect fellowship with the Creator. They are following His Health Plan to the letter.

While it may not be so easy for us today after thousands of years of deception, it is still possible to enjoy the incredible benefits God intended for us. His Health Plan still exists, just waiting to bring healing to our bodies and our minds.

14

THE DEPTH OF THE DECEPTION

"Let me get this straight," David said as I closed the Bible and slid it across the desk in his direction. "You're telling me that if I don't want to have another heart attack, I've got to become a gardener?"

I couldn't help but laugh at his question, even though I sensed a touch of frustration in his voice. "Wouldn't hurt," I responded with a chuckle. "Doesn't pay much, though."

David's eyes narrowed. "Doc," he said. "This Bible—this 'owner's manual' as you call it—just seems to be full of outdated concepts that don't make sense in today's world."

"Oh, really?" I asked. "Then how do you explain that many— if not most—of the diseases with which we struggle today became widespread as more and more of us moved from the country into the cities, as we turned our backs on our farms and became apartment dwellers and factory workers? How do you explain that even today, the healthiest societies are still those in which people work the land and eat their own harvest—people like the rural Chinese,

Japanese, or Southeast Asians? How do you explain the fact that history records the longevity of nations whose people lived off the land—nations like the ancient Mayans or many African societies? Try to find heart disease in today's African backcountries. Try to find diabetes among the poor farming communities of Asia and South America.

"For that matter," I pressed, "look at North America. Before 1900, our diet consisted mostly of foods grown in local gardens and on nearby farms, supplemented with a few choice items from the general store. What meat we did eat on special occasions came from our own barnyard. In 1900, 10 to 15 percent of deaths in the country were from cardiovascular disease. Now, as we move into the twenty-first century—just over one hundred years later—almost every second death is from heart disease. Even cancer deaths have shot up dramatically, in spite of modern medical interventions. David, people didn't change. But our lifestyles did, especially when it comes to what we dumped down our throats. We've moved from kernels of corn to buckets from the "Colonel." We've traded spring water for soda pop. The whole foods nature so willingly provides now have the nutrition processed right out of them, and to make up for the loss of flavor, we pour on sugars, salts, and copious amounts of preservatives to increase shelf life and 'eye appeal.' I stand by my statement. We could all do a lot worse than become gardeners."

David was silent for a long moment. I sensed a crack beginning to form in his outer shell of frustration, so I continued, hoping he would allow a few more pieces of the puzzle to fall into place.

Subtle Dangers

I shared with my patient a short list of risks to his health of which he, and most of my patients, are blissfully unaware. These deceptions are literally killing people. I see it every day. Now let's take a look at the list I gave David.

Deception 1: Caffeine Makes You Think Better

Just the opposite is true. Caffeine binds to receptors in the brain that constrict blood flow. The body, sensing the restriction, responds to the stress with increased adrenaline. This action decreases dopamine in the brain. Dopamine is a neurotransmitter that is naturally produced in the body and is present in the regions of the brain that regulate movement, emotion, motivation, and the feeling of pleasure. This neurotransmitter also stabilizes brain activity *and regulates the flow of information* to other parts of the brain. So, if caffeine decreases dopamine, your thinking isn't going to be any better.

Caffeine is also an addictive substance. That is why so many products have it listed in their ingredients panel. Manufacturers aren't trying to make their product better by doing this. They toss it in there for one reason—to get you addicted so you'll buy more of what they're selling. Pretty clever. (For that matter, just think of all the other chemicals about which we know nothing that are included in lists of ingredients. Why are they there? What are their side effects? What are they doing to our bodies?)

Deception 2: Daylight Saving Time Is a Harmless Energy-Conservation Measure

The October 30, 2008, issue of the *New England Journal of Medicine* reported an increase in heart attacks after daylight saving time was implemented. Why is that? Because when the brain that governs our sleep/awake rhythms is forced to move an hour forward or backward, unneeded stress is placed on the body. You may have noticed this as you try to adjust to the time change each spring and fall. Our body's chemical, electrical, hormonal, and immunologic environments experience stress in adjusting to the change in rest patterns.

There are really few if any benefits from changing the time back and forth, though the politicians sold it as harmless. This twice-a-year ritual increases stress and bumps up heart-attack risk.

Why do we keep doing it? Perhaps stores want us to enjoy a longer shopping day. Perhaps we just want more daylight time to have fun. But we are paying a price for that pleasure.

Deception 3: Sugar Is Good for You

This seems to be the message heralded by many food manufacturers. Look at the ingredients of most of your grocery-store or fast-food favorites, and you'll find sugar or high-fructose corn syrup—or one of sugar's many other chemical equivalents—listed as a major ingredient.

Someone once told me if we taxed corn syrup significantly, we would have no health crisis in this country because obesity levels would decline. But as long as sugar is relatively cheap, it will find its way into most foods.

There is another problem that is anything but sweet. Sugar is addictive. It acts on the brain to make you feel good. Think about it. How many times have you (and I) eaten an entire box of cookies instead of enjoying just one? Were we really that hungry? No. But after a while, receptors in our brains get used to sugar, and it takes more and more to achieve the desired pleasure response. This is a classic example of an addiction under development.

Unfortunately, we're also consuming too many calories, which leads to fat storage and the added stress that extra weight brings to the system. We are being deceived into thinking there are no long-term consequences of eating an entire box of cookies—or chips, or candies, or whatever. Food manufacturers are blatantly and effectively addicting an entire generation. We were not designed to eat this way.

Deception 4: The Bigger the Better

Supersize it! Doing so might achieve a short-term economic gain for a fast-food chain, but in the long run, we are all losers.

Here's a surprising fact. Long-term survival studies indicate that the less we eat, the longer we live. Again, we need to think about how our actions today will affect the future. We really need to be downsizing our food portions unless our diets consist of high-nutrition, high-fiber, whole-plant foods. Only then is it actually possible to eat more and weigh less. But if you eat the standard American diet, watch out. And don't let anyone—especially the fast-food industry—tell you different.

Deception 5: Cow's Milk Is Good for You

I would have to say that of all the deceptions we face, this one leads the pack. Humans are the only mammals who continue to drink milk after the weaning period. We are also the only mammals who drink the milk of another species.

In *The China Study*, T. Colin Campbell provides compelling evidence that milk is far from the healthy beverage advertisers say it is. As a matter of fact, after years of highly scientific research, he made this rather startling conclusion concerning the connection between milk consumption and cancer in tightly controlled laboratory animals: "Casein, which makes up 87% of cow's milk protein, promoted all stages of the cancer process. What type of protein did not promote cancer, even at high levels of intake? The safe proteins were from plants, including wheat and soy" (p. 6). Then he adds, speaking of his now-famous China study, "What made this project especially remarkable is that, among the many associations that are relevant to diet and disease, so many pointed to the same find-ing: people who ate the most animal-based foods got the most chronic disease. Even relatively small intakes of animal-based food were associated with adverse effects. People who ate the most plant-based foods were the healthiest and tended to avoid chronic disease" (p. 7).

Make no mistake about it. Milk is nothing more than liquid meat.

"But what about calcium?" I hear you ask. Milk certainly contains calcium, placed there by the cow's body. We humans manufacture calcium as well. But here's the problem. When we drink cow's milk (or goat's milk), we are introducing an acidic food into our system, because all animal-based foods are acidic. Our bodies, which try to maintain a balanced pH level that favors the alkaline side of the scale, immediately set about attempting to neutralize this newly introduced acid. How do they do this? By applying their best neutralizer. And what is this all-important element that our bodies utilize to tame the acid in the milk? It's the calcium stored in our bones. That's right. Milk doesn't build our bones. Instead, it causes our bodies to leach their own calcium into the bloodstream in order to neutralize the intruder, thus actually *removing* calcium from our bones. Is it any wonder that in countries where the most milk is consumed, we find the greatest rate of osteoporosis?

Why don't we hear about this? Because the milk industry has taken a specific truth—that milk contains calcium—and created a marketing scheme that works to their advantage. We think we are doing something good for our bodies. But we're not. We are liter-ally destroying the very bones the marketers say we are building.

I don't mean to gross you out, but if cows could talk, what would you think if you saw one of those gentle creatures approaching a lactating woman and saying, "Excuse me, lady.

I'm running a little short on milk. May I have some of yours to feed my calf?" In essence, that is exactly what we're doing to the cow. And although the theory has probably never been tested, I'm pretty sure that human milk would be just as unhealthy for the cow as cow's milk is to the human.

This leads us to our next deception.

Deception 6: The Media Tells the Truth and Wants the Best for You

The media can be a powerful tool for good. It can be a terrific vehicle for spreading the truth. I hope you believe that this book is an example of that. But think about it: the media is also all about making money for advertisers.

I have patients come to me asking about miracle substances they've read about in a magazine or discovered on the Internet. Some of these pills, potions, or procedures are harmless. But often, well-meaning individuals spend a lot of money on substances that carry no evidence of being truly beneficial. In fact, sometimes these magical potions do not even have the ingredients they claim to contain. Remember, the Food and Drug Administration does not regulate many of these substances. So there is often no science behind the claims.

That is why I've created what I call the "Marcum Test" when it comes to such products. You might want to consider using such a process when you are facing a health-product decision.

First, I ask myself, "Does this product make sense?" I know enough about the human body to realize that most health problems require several physiological responses, not just one. There's no "magic bullet" when it comes to building and maintaining optimum health. Anything claiming to cure a long list of ills doesn't get much of my attention. Yes, it may do one or two things well, but if it falls all over itself trying to convince you that you've just found the secret for everything that ails you, keep looking.

Second, I want to know, "Is there science behind this?" I'm not talking about a study created by the manufacturer of the product, which serves to prove its marketing claims. I'm talking about hard scientific evidence supporting what the product says it can do.

And third, I ask, "Does this product or concept agree with the owner's manual, the Bible?" Where does it fit in with God's overall Health Plan for our lives?"

Finally I ask, "Is it available to all God's creatures?" God is the ultimate unselfish Being. He makes His "health products" available to all people everywhere.

Deception 7: We Have a National Health Care Crisis

I don't mean to sound unpatriotic, but no government has the solution to health care when it is estimated that 80 percent of disease in that nation or country is lifestyle related. Can you see lawmakers in Washington, DC, telling us how to live our lives? We wouldn't listen. We're far too independent.

Our health care crisis is not national. It's *personal*. In the recently released documentary *Forks over Knives*, T. Colin Campbell suggests it would be possible to reduce health care costs by more than 70 percent if people just changed their diets. This is a personal decision, one that cannot be legislated. The answer has to come from within our own lives and the choices we make every day. Real change must be the result of sound education and clear-headed, unbiased thinking, not of a majority vote.

Deception 8: Someone Is Protecting Us

With more than fourteen thousand chemicals added to the American food supply on a regular basis, how can anyone be sure what these chemicals are doing to us and how they are reacting with other chemicals? The deception is that this practice is actually safe!

Many of these chemicals have absolutely no food value, and some are nothing more than addictive substances tossed in to boost sales. Consider these examples: monosodium glutamate (MSG) and aspartame (an artificial sweetener) have been shown to be toxic to the neurons in young brains. Other food additives gaining attention include benzene (a colorless, volatile, flammable, toxic liquid used in organic synthesis, as a solvent, *and as a motor fuel*); BHA (a phenolic—that is, a disinfectant—antioxidant used especially to preserve fats and oils in food); and anything hydrolyzed (the chemical process of decomposition). This stuff is in our food!

We don't understand how our bodies will react to these toxins over time. But if human history is any template, we are about to find out. We are all becoming laboratory rats in an ongoing study, the results of which I can guarantee you will not be pretty.

That is what I love most about the whole foods God created for us to eat—no chemicals or additives necessary. No preservatives required. Not even a nutrition label needed. Whole foods straight from the hand of God are nutritious, delicious, and tailor made for human consumption. No worries, no dangers, no tricks.

Now that I think about it, I guess I was wrong. Someone *is* protecting us.

The Ripple Effect

Recently, Michelle came into my office suffering from chest pains. The reason for her chest pains is a prime example of what happens when we deviate from God's original ideal for us— when we allow ourselves to live lives that are the result of deception. This is a story you will not soon forget.

For twenty years Michelle served an upscale company as an executive secretary. She told me every day she put on her high-heel shoes and happily headed off to work. Her shoes were expected office attire and reflected the company's image perfectly.

After twenty years, her feet began to have significant problems. There was increasing pain each time she tried to walk, so she made an appointment with a podiatrist who diagnosed the problem and recommended surgery. Because of the persistent pain, she stopped her regular exercise routine. Two operations later, she was still unable to walk comfortably but found some relief from her problems in food. She quickly put on weight, which in time caused her to develop diabetes, hypertension, and sleep apnea. Her doctors placed her on medications and suggested a sleep mask. But Michelle still couldn't rest because of the severe pain in her feet, so she started taking powerful narcotics and a sleeping pill. Subsequently she was replaced at work because her boss said she was not as sharp as she used to be.

The narcotics she was taking slowed down her intestines, and soon she had a bowel obstruction complicated by an infection. She had also developed chest pains, and that is why she came to see me.

When I heard Michelle's tale of woe, I shook my head in amazement. What a horror story! When one stress to the body occurs—even if it occurs slowly—there is often a ripple effect. Michelle might have bypassed this entire cascade of illnesses if she'd simply tossed her high-heel shoes in the dumpster twenty years ago and found a new job that allowed her to wear stylish flats.

When Michelle heard I was writing this book, she asked me to include her story, hoping to get people to think about the consequences of even the simplest actions taken outside of God's design for our lives. Michelle did not realize the damage her choice of footwear had been causing. High heels are not necessarily bad, but in the wrong situation they can be damaging. This concept can apply to the clothes we wear, the chemicals we smear on our bodies to smell or look good, the substances we ingest, the images we dwell on, the sounds we hear—all have an impact on us in what can be dramatic ways. Whether we like it or not, everything we do makes a difference—one way or another—to our health. I believe we owe it to ourselves to think about such things and not blindly follow popular or cultural trends. Doing so just might cause a ripple effect twenty years down the road. Trust me, when we live lives overrun by deceptions, there *will* be ripple effects.

But if you have read this far, you know we have a standard by which to judge every decision we make. We know how we were designed to live. There is no mystery to solve or puzzle to piece together. God made us, understands perfectly what we need to do to stay healthy, and provides the needed elements each and every day of our lives. However, so few learn His principles of health and take advantage of His guidance.

What happened to change our world so profoundly? How did we get from the Garden of Eden to the mess we now call life? The answers to those two questions will form the very foundation of healthy living for you and your family. In the story of earth's most horrible deception, we find both the causes of all disease and the cures for all infirmities. It's also where we will discover the incredible power and eternal benefits of the ultimate prescription.

15

THE LIE

It was a blustery, cold January morning in 2007 when a man made his way to the Metro station in Washington, DC, and took up a position in the bustling lobby. With streams of people passing by, he retrieved a violin from the case he was carrying and began to adeptly tune the strings. Once satisfied that the tones would be perfect and that the hair on the bow was adjusted properly, he lifted the instrument to his chin and began to play.

The notes he created mingled with the shuffling of shoes, the clanking of coins dropping into ticket machines, the clatter of the turnstiles, and the distant rumble of the trains. For forty-five minutes he filled the busy enclosure with intricate trills and the metered melodies of Johann Sebastian Bach, never missing a note. His inflections and emotional renderings were flawless.

While the musician played, one middle-aged man stopped for a moment, then moved on. A few minutes later, a woman tossed a dollar bill into the open violin case as she hurried by.

Several children paused quizzically before being dragged away by preoccupied parents.

After completing his forty-five-minute concert, the man counted up his earnings for the morning. He found thirty-two dollars in his case, placed there by approximately twenty people, none of whom had even stopped to listen. As a matter of fact, no one—save the middle-aged man, with his short visit—had taken the time to enjoy the music.

No one had applauded or shown more than a passing interest in the musician. What they did not know—or even try to discover—was that the man in the lobby was Joshua Bell, one of the world's greatest violinists. The instrument he was playing was valued at more than $3.5 million dollars. Just two days before, this same musician had performed in Boston to a packed concert hall, where tickets averaged a hundred dollars each.

It is evident from this story that at such an unusual time and in such an unusual place, several thousand individuals failed to recognize one of the most talented musicians of our generation playing some of the finest music ever written on one of the most exquisite instruments ever created. They simply didn't stop to listen.

Does this happen to you? Are you too busy, too preoccupied, too overcome with the realities of living on this deceived planet to listen to your Creator talking to you about your health— perhaps at times and places where you would least expect it? If you are, there is a reason. And that reason took root in the Garden of Eden.

The Voice in the Tree

Much had already taken place in the universe before Adam and Eve began walking the lush paths of their beautiful Garden. According to Scripture, one of God's most talented and wise creations, an angel named Lucifer, had become disenchanted with how things were. Bible scholars agree that this special being felt he was not being given the attention he deserved, so he started a rumor campaign against God, telling the other created beings how he—and they—were nothing more than subjects under the thumb of a heartless dictator.

To make a long story short, Lucifer, who is also called "the dragon" in the Bible, finally gained enough followers and stirred up enough trouble that God felt compelled to take action. Here's how John the revelator described what happened next: "There was war in heaven. Michael and his angels fought against the dragon and his angels. And the dragon lost the battle, and he and his angels were forced out of heaven. This great dragon—the ancient serpent called the devil, or Satan, the one deceiving the whole world—was thrown down to the earth with all his angels" (Revelation 12:7-9).

Referring to this event—and Satan's eventual destruction—as well as providing a tiny glimpse into the motivation behind Satan's rebellion, the Old Testament prophet Isaiah writes,

> *How you are fallen from heaven,*
> *O shining star, son of the morning!*
> *You have been thrown down to the earth,*
> *you who destroyed the nations of the world.*
> *For you said to yourself,*
> *"I will ascend to heaven and set my throne*
> *above God's stars.*
> *I will preside on the mountain of the gods*
> *far away in the north.*
> *I will climb to the highest heavens*
> *and be like the Most High."*
> *Instead, you will be brought down to the place of the dead,*
> *down to its lowest depths.* (Isaiah 14:12-15)

Satan sure used the word *I* a lot, didn't he? He was all about what *he* wanted, what *he* was trying to accomplish, what made *him* feel good about himself. We might even call him selfish. God, on the other hand, is unfailingly concerned about others, about you . . . and about me. He is focused on us, on *our* well-being. Is it any wonder that two such opposing factions could not coexist within the perfect harmony of heaven?

So Satan lost his exalted position in the presence of God and ended up in the only place in the universe where he would not be immediately expelled by the inhabitants—our brand-new, virtually unpopulated earth. And that is where he appeared as a serpent to Eve one day.

We pick up the story in Genesis 3:1: "The serpent was the shrewdest of all the wild animals the LORD God had made. One day he asked the woman, 'Did God really say you must not eat the fruit from any of the trees in the garden?'"

First of all, we must remember that God had indeed conversed with Adam concerning the very tree in which the serpent now sprawled. He had told Adam, "You may freely eat the fruit of every tree in the garden—except the tree of the knowledge of good and evil. If you eat its fruit, you are sure to die" (Genesis 2:16-17).

Eve must have been aware of this command, because she calmly answered the serpent, "Of course we may eat fruit from the trees in the garden. . . . It's only the fruit from the tree in the middle of the garden that we are not allowed to eat. God said, 'You must not eat it or even touch it; if you do, you will die'" (Genesis 3:2-3).

What happened next is still having an impact on our lives today. The words Satan spoke in response to Eve's statement form the very core of our present health crises, our spiritual detachments, our relationship struggles, and our many mental diseases. I can imagine the serpent lowering himself to eye level with the woman, smiling reassuringly, and saying in a soothing, confident voice, "You won't die! . . . God knows that your eyes will be opened as soon as you eat it, and you will be like God, knowing both good and evil" (Genesis 3:4-5).

You won't die. Go ahead. Eat the forbidden fruit; choose whatever you want; enjoy all the junk food your heart desires; completely ignore your circadian rhythm; fill your mind with scenes of sex and violence; destroy God's creatures to satisfy your perverted appetite; stare at a computer terminal all day; text instead of talk; ride instead of walk; lust instead of love; worship technology, sports, and anything else except the true God; none of those things will hurt you. What does God know? He's a heartless dictator who just wants you to be His slave and do exactly what He says or . . . well . . . look what happened to me. I got tossed out of heaven because I dared confront Him with the truth.

You won't die. Millions of people still believe those words when they light up their first cigarette, make food choices based solely on what satisfies their additive-perverted taste buds, hurry past nutrition-packed foods in the grocery store as they load their shopping carts with highly processed favorites. How many people shuffle off to the doctor's office seeking answers to their illnesses when, like Eve, the garden in which they live overflows with what they really need to build and maintain optimum health?

The same serpent that deceived Eve about the fruit of that long-forgotten tree still moves in the shadows of our lives today, ready to repeat his deadly declaration in our times of indecision: "You won't die!"

God's words to Adam and Eve were more than a warning. They were identifying a set of laws—the very same laws that hold the universe in place. God's revelation also specified in no uncertain terms what would happen if those laws were broken. Death, and the self-imposed sicknesses that often result in death, are not punishments from God. The fact that Adam and Eve—and every generation since—have passed away is not because God is punishing anyone for breaking His laws. If you jump out of an airborne plane without a parachute, you will die, not because God is unhappy with you but because breaking certain laws brings about certain consequences. When God told Adam that if he ate of the forbidden fruit he would die, he wasn't bringing judgment down on the man's head. He was simply allowing earth's first humans to make a choice based on complete and proper information. Don't eat that fruit, and you live forever. Eat the fruit, and you die. Period.

When God spoke to Adam, He was identifying a choice between two paths to follow—one based on universal law, the other based on life lived outside that law. The latter is where Satan had chosen to spend his existence. In essence, God was saying, "Adam, Eve, here's the deal. My laws, based on love and liberty, will lead to eternal life. You can walk with me, talk face-to-face with me, and enjoy all the benefits of living in harmony with my universal laws. But I'm no dictator. I know that love without liberty is not love at all. So I give you the ability to choose. You can determine your own future. You can decide which path you want to follow. The tree of which I am speaking represents everything that is not within my path. I put it there so that you can demonstrate to me—and all created beings—that you *choose* to remain loyal to my laws of love. You have to understand that by eating the fruit of that tree, you will be switching paths, and the consequence of doing so will mean eternal separation from me. You . . . will . . . die."

The power of choice—the most amazing and dangerous gift God ever bestowed on humankind—is a product of love, not dominion.

Christian psychiatrist and author Dr. Timothy Jennings in his book *Could It Be This Simple?* puts it this way: "It is impossible for love to exist in an atmosphere without freedom. If you're not sure, try it on your spouse. Tell him or her that if they don't love you, you will kill them. Restrict your spouse's liberties, and see what then happens to love. The law of liberty is one of the cornerstone principles of God's government. As God is love, He necessarily *must* respect the liberty and individuality of His intelligent creatures. To do otherwise would destroy love and incite rebellion" (Autumn House, 2007, p. 49).

It was safely within this very liberty that Eve walked in the Garden that day. It was because of this liberty that the serpent was able to spew his verbal venom on such an innocent woman. And it was within the boundaries of that liberty that Eve did the unthinkable. "The woman was convinced. She saw that the tree was beautiful and its fruit looked delicious, and she wanted the wisdom it would give her. So she took some of the fruit and ate it. Then she gave some to her husband, who was with her, and he ate it, too" (Genesis 3:6).

Later in the Old Testament, King Solomon stated what by then should have been totally obvious to everyone: "There is a path before each person that seems right, but it ends in death" (Proverbs 14:12).

Two paths—one comfortably within God's law of love, the other outside that law. Two results—one future designed by the loving mind of a Creator God, the other constructed by a mind filled with rebellion and self-interest. Adam and Eve chose the second path, and we are still stumbling along its rugged and dangerous outline today. This second path has led to ongoing deception, causing stress on the system, including our very own DNA and the resultant change in chemistry. This then leads to symptoms and a need for modern medicine.

But—and here's the best news any cardiologist or health practitioner can give to a patient—that first path still exists! The laws that govern it, shape it, and determine its destination still wait for all those who choose to turn their backs on the lies of Satan. Only along *this* path can we find optimum health. Only on the path created by love do we find the answers to our most troubling health questions. Contrary to what Satan has been saying for thousands of years, it is *only* on this path that we can find the whole, unblemished truth about how to overcome disease and—even more important—reestablish our lost connection with the God who created us.

Eden set the standard for gaining and maintaining optimal physical health. Within those seven days of Creation, we discovered the powerful laws that govern the well-being of every creature on earth. But there was another element in Satan's statement to Eve that is just as destructive to minds and bodies as the belief that God's laws were not really put in place for our ultimate good. If you read between the lines, you will uncover a frightening undercurrent in which many struggle to this day. What so few realize is that this undercurrent—this hidden message—can make us very, very sick.

16

THE PATH OF TRUTH

IN HIS FASCINATING BOOK *Cheating Death*, Dr. Sanjay Gupta, a neurosurgeon, deftly describes many situations in which the end of life is delayed or completely avoided—at least for the time being. Dr. Gupta, who has been described as "The World's Doctor," brings to light many instances where technology has progressed to the point where it can actually, in his words, "cheat death." This amazing technology includes utilizing the effects of hypothermia, applying more aggressive resuscitation techniques, introducing such elements as hydrogen sulfide into trauma victims' bodies to slow metabolism, and performing delicate procedures on unborn babies to correct birth defects, fetal tumors, urinary blockages, and hernias of the diaphragm. These new technological advances can save lives where at one time modern medicine had nothing to offer.

What this new technology is doing is "buying time" so further healing can take place, either through modern medicine or through the body's own ability to eventually fix what is wrong.

While we mere mortals can't understand all aspects of healing, God has given us the intelligence to apply His powerful laws of health even though we may not fully comprehend how they work. It underscores for me the fact that our Great Physician—the God who made us—is truly at the center of every healing encounter and should be part of every treatment plan. The One who makes it all possible should lead modern medicine. Only through His power and intervention can we truly "cheat" death.

Which brings up a question: in the midst of the worldwide health crisis in which we find ourselves today, why are we not hearing more about God's original Health Plan? People like David need surgeries, medications, and are sicker than ever before. There is real suffering all around. One would think something needs to change, and the sooner the better. We in the healing world are missing something. Why are we not looking for a new approach? Why are we not looking at the real cause of the problem?

I must admit that modern technology is exciting and the ability to "cheat" death is dramatic. I enjoy the medical dramas too, but how did we get in a position of almost total disconnect with our Master Healer in the first place? Why have we moved so far from the original plan? If we understand why this has happened to our world, perhaps we can rediscover the balance in healing.

I think it's high time to tell what the late broadcaster Paul Harvey called "the rest of the story." The rest of the story will answer the question why. Just as there is a reason for every illness, there is a reason why we are searching for healing in all the wrong places. There is a deception out there of which many are unaware.

Deeper Antagonism

I firmly believe that the foundation for our self-imposed ignorance is found in the Garden of Eden where a beguiling serpent spoke to Adam and Eve one day. As we have already discovered, his words reverberated from a heart darkened by self-interest and rebellion. He not only insisted that God was not telling the truth, but he also revealed a deeper antagonism for the Creator. In a voice soothing yet provoking, Satan implied that God wasn't who He said He was. There was no love in Satan's actions. He was challenging the true nature of God. Who would want a God like the one Satan described to be in charge of healing?

I like the illustration that my colleague, Dr. Timothy Jennings, shares with many of his patients when he and they are discussing the subject of love and trust. He asks them to consider this scenario: Someone you know tells you that your spouse has been cheating on you. He or she even presents false evidence—digitally altered photographs showing your husband or wife in compromising positions with another person. How do you feel about your spouse after receiving that information? The fact that your husband or wife is totally innocent of wrongdoing means nothing *if you believe the lie*. And if you do, does your relationship with him or her change? Do you find it hard to trust your spouse? Do you believe anything he or she says from that moment on?

Then Dr. Jennings drives home the story with these words: "Lies believed break the circle of love and trust. This leads to a spirit of fear, selfishness, and rebellion."

Sound familiar? I think it's safe to say that Satan ran a highly successful rumor campaign against God. His lies—that God was an enslaving dictator with little regard for the "little people" in His heavenly Kingdom—convinced a lot of angels to rebel, even though there was not a grain of truth in Satan's arguments. Why do I bring this up? Because unless we understand the problem and its origin, we do not have a chance of finding the solution. This original deception—that God cannot be trusted—and the subsequent lies about His character were the real problems. This set up a cascade of events we are still a part of today.

Now we find this same deceiver facing Adam and Eve in the Garden, and from his mouth issues the same venom that got him booted out of heaven. The statement "You won't die!" was meant to cast doubt on God's honesty and integrity. Then Satan added this devastating punch line: "God knows that your eyes will be opened as soon as you eat it, and you will be like God, knowing both good and evil" (Genesis 3:5).

The serpent was right—to a point. Once Adam and Eve had disobeyed a direct command from God—do not eat from that tree—their eyes were certainly open to knowing good and evil. They had known good, but *now* they also knew the unsettling discomfort of having done evil.

It's the statement "You will be like God" that caused the most devastating rift between the Creator and His two freshly minted humans. Suddenly, in their minds, God was not the perfect Being filled with unselfish love and wise counsel. If they were now "like God," that meant that He must be flawed, self-seeking, and prone to doubt, just as they were feeling inside. In other words, in their minds, God's character had changed. Because they had believed the lie and disobeyed, the circle of love and trust was broken, and their precious Creator was now someone they did not trust. Very quickly that mistrust turned to fear. The deception was taking root and beginning to grow. Why should we believe the Health Plan or anything this type of untrustworthy God recommends?

False God

If I were to say to my patient David, "I routinely violate God's original plan. It is just impossible for me to follow," this would cast doubt as to whether it is humanly possible for David, or anyone else for that matter, to follow the original template. God's plan for the universe isn't unreasonable. But as we fall into deceptions, we gradually become enslaved in them. "See?" the devil exults as we find ourselves irresistibly attracted to sin and helplessly enslaved to it, "I *told* you there was something wrong with God's way! *No one* can live up to His expectations!" This is exactly where Adam and Eve found themselves, and we wonder why God's Health Plan isn't getting any attention.

"But, Dr. Marcum," I can hear you saying, "I don't believe Satan's lies about God!"

I'm so thankful for those people who make that claim, because this means they are truly trying to serve the God they love. But then I must ask a very pointed and, in some circles, highly controversial question. "Is the God you love and worship the true God or one based on lies—falsehoods of which you may not even be aware?" Are you worshiping God or a being society has created? Think about this for a few minutes. This is important. Allow me to provide some examples of this horrible lie.

Most Christians worship a god who, in essence, says, "I love you so much. I created the world for you and died on the cross for you, and I will someday come and take you home to live with me in heaven forever and ever. However, if you break my commandments or turn your back on my love, I will kill you."

Think long and hard about what I just said. Is that your God? Believing in such a "fire and brimstone" heavenly Father might provide a strong motivation for obedience, but it hardly creates a comfortable foundation on which to build a loving relationship.

There's more. Continuing our Genesis story, we read what happened after Adam and Eve's encounter with the serpent: "When the cool evening breezes were blowing, the man and his wife heard the LORD God walking about in the garden. So they hid from the LORD God among the trees. Then the LORD God called to the man, 'Where are you?'

"He replied, 'I heard you walking in the garden, so I hid'" (Genesis 3:8-10).

Afraid? Of God? Why?

"'I was afraid because I was naked.'

"'Who told you that you were naked?' the LORD God asked. 'Have you eaten from the tree whose fruit I commanded you not to eat?'" (vv. 10-11).

There's something interesting here. Adam's sin had apparently stripped him of the divine glory that had "clothed" both him and Eve, a covering that allowed them to feel completely at ease in the presence of their Creator. They were now uncomfortable. This was not part of the original plan. Once again I am reminded of Dr. Jennings's words: "Lies believed break the circle of love and trust. This leads to a spirit of fear, selfishness, and rebellion."

Then God asked Adam, "Who told you that you were naked?" (v. 11). Wait a minute! It seems God was not the force generating the grinding guilt that created Adam's fear. Adam and Eve felt guilty—and naked—even before the Lord showed up. I believe what they were feeling was the uncertainty and dread that come from walking the path prepared by Satan. They were off course. Something wasn't right. For the first time, they were experiencing the stress that comes from living outside the protective presence of their Creator. Their chemistry was changing— and not for the good. They had placed themselves firmly on the wrong path—the path that according to God leads to death.

Notice that this death is a result of sin. God simply allows Adam and Eve to reap the consequences of walking the path that leads to eternal separation from Him.

When Adam and Eve discovered the Lord was nearby, they hid in the bushes. After all, the God who had made them must be a vengeful God. Didn't He throw Satan and his followers out of heaven simply because they dared to disagree with Him?

Do you see the change taking place here? God had done no wrong, but Adam and Eve believed Satan's lies, and lies believed change everything. Are we running and hiding from our true Healer? Does it make any sense to run from love? Has the world told us how to think of and relate to God? Are we operating from a true and accurate picture of Him?

The Woman

Let's spend a moment in the New Testament exploring another popular misconception of our heavenly Father. We find a revealing story in the book of John. A group of self-righteous and very "religious" men come before Jesus dragging with them a woman who had been "caught in the act of adultery." "Teacher," they say, shoving their victim down at Christ's feet, "the law of Moses says to stone her. What do you say?" (see John 8:4-5).

According to John's account, Jesus "stooped down and wrote in the dust with his finger. They kept demanding an answer, so he stood up again and said, 'All right, but let the one who has never sinned throw the first stone!' Then he stooped down again and wrote in the dust" (vv. 6-8).

I am not sure what Jesus wrote on the ground—perhaps street addresses or people's names—but whatever information he scratched in the dirt made an impression, because one by one the woman's accusers decided they had important business elsewhere. Finally, only Jesus and the woman remained.

Now listen carefully to what Jesus said to her and see if it matches your concept of the God you worship—especially when you come to Him from deep in sin. "Jesus stood up again and said to the woman, 'Where are your accusers? Didn't even one of them condemn you?'

"'No, Lord,' she said.

"And Jesus said, 'Neither do I. Go and sin no more'" (vv. 10-11).

According to this account, the condemnation we feel when we have sinned is not from God. Here was a woman caught *in the act* of adultery. There was no question she was breaking one of the Ten Commandments. But Christ—who was fully aware of this—said He did not condemn her. Instead, He told her essentially, "What you were doing is a sin, so stop doing it!" No judgment, no dire warning of impending punishment, no thunderous sermons about hellfire, no unyielding demand for repentance, no condemnation. But you know what? I have a feeling that the woman, fresh from the arms of a married man who wasn't her husband, found something unexpected that day. She discovered a type of love that turns fearful sinners into thankful, adoring worshipers. She found, at the feet of Jesus, an acceptance that no church, no society, no culture had ever offered her. For the first time she caught a glimpse of the real God, the true God, from whom humankind had been hiding since Adam and Eve ate the fruit from the forbidden tree, since they switched paths from God's way to Satan's way and took the whole world with them. That woman, like so many of us, had believed a lie. Now she was looking directly into the face of absolute truth, and it transformed her. Her chemistry was changing. Healing had begun.

Maybe you're thinking, *Yeah, well, when you're dealing with Jesus, that's one thing. But God the Father, watch out! He's the judge, jury, and executioner all rolled into one.*

Really? Listen to what Jesus said when one of His disciples asked him a very direct question during what we call "The Last Supper."

Christ has just made the statement "No one can come to the Father except through me." This was followed by "If you had really known me, you would know who my Father is. From now on, you do know him and have seen him!" (John 14:6-7).

Here's what happened next: "Philip said, 'Lord, show us the Father, and we will be satisfied.'

"Jesus replied: 'Have I been with you all this time, Philip, and yet you still don't know who I am? Anyone who has seen me has seen the Father! So why are you asking me to show him to you? Don't you believe that I am in the Father and the Father is in me? The words I speak are not my own, but my Father who lives in me does his work through me'" (vv. 8-10). God was dispelling the deceptions and revealing the truth of what love looked like through His Son. This was His character. He was not at all like the portrait painted by Satan. Here was proof.

If I were to ask you, "Who would you rather have judge you at the end of time, Jesus or God the Father?" I have a feeling that many would say, "Give me Jesus!" Why? Because so many of us think of God the Father as a harsh, demanding judge with whom Jesus is pleading our case, asking for lenience for us poor, ignorant sinners. Where did *that* come from?

It came from Eden. It came from the branches of the tree of the knowledge of good and evil. It came from the mouth of the master deceiver, Satan. Jesus and His Father are one in thought, one in action, and one in their determination to bring saving love into every life. They long to heal. The reason we are not being drawn to God as the Master Healer, to the Great Physician, and to His Health Plan lies in the deceptions passed down from generation to generation.

Apart from God

I could go on and on, but I won't. There are many resources available to help you on this journey to a clearer and more realistic picture of our heavenly Father. But I have brought you to this point for a reason. We are trying to discover why we have departed from the original Health Plan given at Creation. Simply put, we have been deceived regarding the nature of God, and now we fear Him instead of love Him. Since Eden, we have been moving further and further from the God who made us. We've been traveling down the slippery slopes of self-worship and dependence on our own intelligence to right our wrongs, bring meaning to our lives, and heal our bodies. We have been carried here on the wings of the greatest deception of all—that God really is not our friend, our guide, our hope. And when we lose hope, we feel alone in this world. When we harbor an unspoken fear of the God of the universe, we introduce stress into our bodies. We change the chemistry that keeps us healthy.

We were designed to worship and love the true God, the God who is love. When this does not occur, we allow fear to drive us into destructive habits and empty relationships. Each of these conditions eats away at our minds, bodies, and spirits the way cancer eats away at muscle, bone, and flesh.

But there is a prescription—an antidote—for this condition. I have seen it work time and time again. It's available to all people everywhere, and it doesn't cost a penny. You just have to know where to find it.

17

THE ULTIMATE PRESCRIPTION

DAVID LOOKED AT ME with questioning eyes. "So, I can do anything I want, and God will still love me?"

I thought for a moment before I responded. "The answer to your question is . . . yes. God is in the loving business, not the condemning business. He's all about life, not death."

My patient had made a remarkable recovery from his heart attack. For months now, he had been doing his best to follow the health guidelines revealed in our owner's manual, the Bible. He had learned to enjoy whole food—foods as grown— and traded his daily sugar-filled soda pops for glasses of pure, refreshing water. He had taken up walking with his wife each day, said good-bye to late-night television so he could get more sleep, and even started observing the weekly rest day God declared holy during Creation. David was feeling great, looking amazing—compared to when I had first seen him—and admitted that he had more energy than ever. I noticed on his chart that his weight was dropping and rejoiced with him when test results revealed no new plaque building up in his arteries. He was experiencing firsthand the incredible power of God's Health Plan.

But I also knew there was more to gaining optimum health than doing all the right things physically. The body and mind are connected in some very powerful ways, and a stressed mind can alter the body's chemistry just as a stressed body can wreak havoc on the mind. If I wanted David to fully recover and live a long, productive life, I would have to make sure there was nothing causing undue tension on his *brain*. This is the one area of recovery many physicians miss or simply ignore.

"Dr. Marcum, you've got to help me understand this," David pressed. "Stress can originate in the brain?"

"Yes, David. When we have misconceptions concerning God. This can take us away from the relationship God intended for us to have with Him. This causes stress. There are definitely evil forces among us—real evil that is destructive and deadly. These evil forces produce counterfeits for God's perfect Health Plan we've been talking about and lead us to sin." I picked up my Bible and thumbed through the pages. "Here's how the Bible identifies it: 'Everyone who sins is breaking God's law, for all sin is contrary to the law of God' (1 John 3:4). And where does this sin lead? 'The wages of sin is death' (Romans 6:23). Sin pulls us away from God's plan.

"So there's definitely sin in this world. But did you notice something interesting here? The apostle Paul, the writer of the letter to the Romans, describes death as a 'wage' of sin. A wage isn't a condemnation. It's payment for services rendered. If you sin, you're paid with death. Then the text continues: 'But the free gift of God is eternal life through Christ Jesus our Lord.' This passage identifies those two paths I talked about earlier—Satan's path and God's path. It also reveals just where those two paths lead—one to life, the other to death. So if you're following Satan's path and you end up dead, did God just zap you with His condemnation, or did you simply reach your destination?

"David, I've found that sin doesn't need a judge to bring punishment to those who live by Satan's rules. As I've said before, sin is self-destructive. It does a very thorough job of ruining lives, breaking hearts, and raining down hurt and agony on those who choose to follow Satan's path. I guess you could say sin is self-judging. It's its own prosecutor, and executioner as well. You're a prime example of what I'm talking about."

David frowned. "You calling me a sinner?"

"Yes, I am." I smiled and added, "Welcome to the club. According to the Bible, we're all sinners living in a sinful world. But God's path runs right through this sinful planet. It's available for any foot to follow. I'm happy to say that's the path you're walking on right now. When you are in a relationship with Him, you are on His path as designed. How does it feel?"

David grinned shyly. "Feels great."

I continued. "While you were walking on Satan's path, you broke some very important health laws. You ate huge amounts of nutritionally empty junk food, lived a sedentary life, and allowed the stresses of everyday living to overpower you. So was your heart attack a judgment from God? No. It was the result of breaking those health laws. These health laws may also have been broken generations ago, and the genetics were passed down to you.

"I tell you this because many people believe that God is a stern judge just waiting to see us fail so He can pronounce a sentence on us. That attitude not only separates us even further from our heavenly Father, but it also totally affects our health. This is the brain stress I have been talking about."

Rearview Mirror

"Have you ever been driving in your car and suddenly noticed in your rearview mirror that a police car is following you? If you're like me, you instantly become the best driver on earth. You nail the speed limit, use your turn signals appropriately, and keep your tires between the lines like never before. Why do you do that?" I asked David.

David chuckled. "I don't want to get caught breaking the law."

"Are you feeling relaxed, happy, contented?"

"No way! I'm feeling tense."

"Even though you're doing everything right?"

"Well . . . yeah!"

"Okay. Let's say you make a turn, and the police car follows you. You make another turn, and that car remains on your tail. How are you feeling now?"

David laughed. "Let's just say I'm trying to figure out whether my registration is up to date, whether my license has expired, whether I have any unpaid parking tickets, and if my insurance check was mailed in on time last month. In other words, I'm a mess."

"So," I pressed, "you're doing absolutely nothing wrong, yet you're completely stressed out over what that police car is doing back there and what the officer might think of you—or know about you?"

My patient nodded. "Yep. That's about right," he said.

"David, that's how many people feel about God. They feel He's back there, following them, ready to pounce, ready to condemn, ready to toss them straight into hell. They live their lives in a state of stress and worry. More to the point, they live their lives in fear—fear of the one source that can bring true healing to their minds, bodies, and spirits. Satan knows that as long as you live in fear, you can't enjoy optimum health. That's why he planted his unfair, untrue, and totally unsubstantiated image of God in Adam's and Eve's minds. He understood that fear is an incredibly powerful stressor, capable even of undoing the good things we do for ourselves.

"Fear has many names—worry, guilt, uncertainty, anger. As long as we fail to grasp the true nature and character of God, our hearts will harbor hidden fear. That's not healthy, nor was it part of God's original plan. When our minds are stressed, our bodies follow this lead chemically.

"But God is not the condemning judge Satan wants us to believe He is. He's something far different."

"Well, then," said David, "what is He?"

"Do you know who Lance Armstrong is?"

My patient blinked. "God is a world-class bicycle racer?"

"Uh, no." I grinned and asked, "When Lance Armstrong races in a tournament, what does he usually have following him?"

"All the other racers?"

"Well, yes, but I'm thinking about the car."

"The car?"

"There's always a little car following him wherever he goes."

"Oh, you mean his support team."

"That's right. And are the people in that car there to record his mistakes, criticize his judgment, and make him feel bad when he does something wrong?"

"No," David interrupted, "they're there to help him fix his bicycle if it breaks, offer assistance if he's injured, and shout encouragement."

"That's right," I said. "David, God is like the support team in that little car. He's following us through life not to condemn but to help. And here's what's really cool about this whole thing. God faithfully follows us no matter which of the two paths we happen to be on."

My patient sat in silence for a long moment. I could see the wheels turning as thoughts he had never entertained sprang to his mind. He was beginning to see an accurate picture of the face of God. Like the woman at Christ's feet, David was beginning to encounter the ultimate prescription.

"David," I continued, "the same God who created laws to help us build and maintain optimum physical health also set in place laws that allow our brains—our thoughts—to become healthy. Those laws are tied directly into how we perceive God. As long as we fear Him—the way we fear the police officer following us—we can never enjoy optimum health of mind *or* body. It's not possible, because our minds have so much influence over our bodies.

"And if we're afraid of Him, we're a lot less willing to believe Him. Suddenly, those health laws He set in place in Eden become nothing more than outdated ancient rituals with little or no relevance to us today. We turn from the Creator to our own understanding or to modern medical practices as our go-to source for health information and guidance. This places us firmly on Satan's path, and we begin a journey that leads to eternal death instead of eternal life. God doesn't condemn us for our choices. But we have a very hard time letting the truth get through to us. But God never quits trying. He is always following in that car."

I studied my patient carefully. "When you go to the store, walk the halls of your office building, or even sit in church, what do you see? Healthy people who are managing their weight correctly, controlling their blood sugar and blood pressure, and taking the moral high ground in life? Or do you see people lost in confusion, desperately depending on the latest wonder drug or high-tech procedure to bring quality back into their lives?"

"It doesn't look very good out there, Doc," David admitted.

"That's because so many need the prescription I'm about to share with you—a medicine so powerful, so overwhelming, that sickness and disease, anger and resentment, fear and uncertainty can't survive for long in its presence. It's hands down the most amazing antidote available on earth. Would you like to know what it is?"

My patient nodded. "Bring it on, Dr. Marcum!"

A Window of Opportunity

The moment was right. My patient David had opened the door, and I was ready for him.

Making people whole again after they have experienced a heart attack depends on several factors: the amount of damage the heart attack has done to the heart, the body's response to the various medicines and procedures that are introduced, the patient's willingness to follow instructions given by his or her cardiologist and recovery team, and just how serious that patient is about regaining health once the acute stage has passed. The damage to David's heart was minimal, owing to the fact that when the attack reached a climax, he was sitting in an emergency room talking to a cardiologist. Most people aren't that fortunate.

When it comes to heart attacks, timing is everything. The window of opportunity for receiving lifesaving help is not measured in days or hours. It's measured in minutes—sometimes seconds.

There is another window of opportunity that opens for a short period of time once patients are out of danger and back home again. They have been frightened by their experience and are willing to make some changes. It is during these few short months—sometimes even weeks—when I try to make my case concerning the true source of health.

Far too many times I have seen patients return to my office and stumble across the threshold—people like David whom my team and I have brought back from the brink of death—with the very same problems developing in their bodies that brought them to me in the first place. Why does this happen? Because they did not address the cause of the original problem. They did not change their lifestyle to accommodate their altered condition. Believe me, if you have survived bypass surgery, you've been altered.

As I said before, nothing is "fixed" by the experience. Patients have simply been handed a second chance, and I praise God for the science behind our ability to accomplish that. But so many patients simply go back to the same old foods, the same old television watching, the same old worries and anxieties, and the same old lack of desire to do the sometimes-hard work necessary to keep them healthy. They don't want to change their lives. They just want me to make them strong enough so they can go back to living as they did before. Pharmaceutical companies depend heavily on this type of patient. The last thing they want these men and women to do is die—or get well. Unfortunately, some medical professionals march under the same banner.

But God calls us—all of us—to be healers, and that includes me. He wants us to come back to the original Health Plan. And if I know the true source of healing, I am going to share the information, even if doing so puts a dent in some drug company's bottom line.

One More Shot

Just before Jesus' betrayal and crucifixion, He was enjoying a final meal with His beloved disciples. He had just sent Judas away and was now left with eleven followers in the upper room. Christ understood that He had only one more shot at getting through to these men before the storm of His arrest, mock trial, and execution swept through their lives.

Summoning their attention, He called out, "Now I am giving you a new commandment" (John 13:34). The disciples—as Jews—understood and obeyed the Ten Commandments that had been handed down at Mount Sinai to their ancestors—rules and regulations that would forever identify them as children of the one true God. But now Christ was facing people very different from the ex-slaves fresh out of Egyptian bondage. He was now talking to "modern" men, well versed in the "how to" of their ancient faith. From this moment on, each disciple would need something more than a set of rules to follow. Jesus knew they were about to need a great deal of healing.

Christ continued. "Love each other. Just as I have loved you, you should love each other" (v. 34). This was the voice of God speaking.

Knowing and obeying a set of rules and regulations were not enough. Doing good was not enough. Preaching well wasn't enough. These eleven men needed to take the next step in their journey to wholeness. They needed to love.

This concept wasn't new in Christ's ministry. When a rich young man came to see Jesus and asked, "What should I do to inherit eternal life?" (Luke 18:18), Christ, at first, took the traditional line. "You know the commandments: 'You must not commit adultery. You must not murder. You must not steal. You must not testify falsely. Honor your father and mother' (v. 20).

"The man replied, 'I've obeyed all these commandments since I was young'" (v. 21).

That's when Jesus added that important, missing element. "There is still one thing you haven't done," He told His visitor. "Sell all your possessions and give the money to the poor, and you will have treasure in heaven. Then come, follow me" (v. 22).

The young man's reaction spoke volumes. "When the man heard this he became very sad, for he was very rich" (v. 23).

What the rich young man lacked was love—love for those without riches, love for those who didn't have the opportunities he enjoyed, love for the "little people" who swarmed about him day in and day out. While being wealthy is certainly no sin, making money and the accumulation of things the determining factor in every decision you make certainly opens the door to selfishness and greed.

But why love? Why is it so important? What did Christ know about it?

I'm not an ordained minister. I haven't studied at the best schools of religion or delved deeply into the ancient texts and the spiritual writings that fill the libraries of theological seminaries.

But I do know a thing or two about medicine and the human body. As I have studied health in general and the heart in particular, I have discovered something incredible. *Love is a healing force*. It can often do what no medicine, procedure, or natural remedy can do. I have seen it in action far too many times to dismiss it simply as an emotion. And I'm not just talking about *being* loved. I am talking about maintaining a loving attitude and *giving* love.

What Is Love?

How do we define such an important concept as love? "It's putting someone else's interest before your own," some say. "God is love," others insist. But I have my own illustration that defines—in small part—what love means to me.

When I come home from a long session at work, no matter what the hour or what worries may be weighing on my mind, my two dogs, Max and Daphne, greet me at the door. You would think they hadn't seen me for months! They are simply beside themselves with joy and eagerly follow me around, just waiting for me to respond to their overflow of emotion. Those with pets can relate to this. Even if, when I left that morning, I'd punished them for something they'd done, like make a mess on the floor or scratch a hole in the screen door, all is forgotten in their unrestrained joy at my return.

You know what? The sight of those two mutts eagerly waiting for me at the door does something to me deep inside. For a moment at least, the worries that were crowding my mind vanish. My weariness fades. My facial muscles automatically pull my lips into a happy smile. From an emotional standpoint, I'm feeling pretty good. But I also know that throughout my body, chemical changes are taking place and bringing health and healing to every cell. That's right. My dogs are helping to bring healing to my heart, my bones, my organs, my blood—all of me. Their unconditional, no-holds-barred love is lowering my stress levels, decreasing my heart rate, dilating my blood vessels, and relaxing my mind in ways no single drug can boast.

I must hasten to add that seeing my two children at the door or catching a glimpse of my beautiful wife walking down the hall does the same thing, but because I work many strange hours, my family is often fast asleep when I return home. Nevertheless, love is an unbelievably powerful prescription.

Love is like that. It's overpowering. It bypasses stress and worry and injects incredible amounts of healing energy into the human body. Endless tests using very sophisticated devices have recorded its profound effect on the mind, body, and spirit of countless individuals. It's no surprise to me when people say, "The moment I fell in love, the sky was bluer, the grass was greener, and even the air smelled wonderful." If they could look inside themselves, they would have also noticed an entire cascade of physiological events taking place, changes that lowered their blood pressure, increased oxygen to the brain, reduced dangerous inflammation, and raised their immune system to new heights.

All these benefits were taking place because they were giving and receiving love.

But love is not something added to human existence to help fight disease. Love was here long before any of God's creation was brought into being. Love is the governing power behind all creation. It drives the unseen machinery of the universe and makes possible all the laws that hold it in place. How do we know this? Because of an amazing text found in the Bible. Think of the implications for your life as you read it. "Anyone who does not love does not know God, for God is love" (1 John 4:8).

This Bible writer doesn't say that God loves or that God needs to be loved. He simply states that God *is* love. That means our heavenly "team" (God the Father, God the Son, and God the Holy Spirit) functions from a foundation of love. Everything they say, everything they do, and every plan they make springs from a well of pure, undefiled love. God cannot operate any other way. Keep this fact in mind the next time you sit down to read your Bible. It will transform your understanding of God's Word and His place in your life.

So if love governs the universe, and love was the driving force behind the creation of this world, should it surprise us that love is a healing element in our lives? We were built for love. We're also maintained by love. And it will be love that sustains us for all eternity.

Further proof of this is demonstrated when love is lost. It is common knowledge among cardiologists that when a loved one dies suddenly, a perfectly healthy spouse can experience surges in epinephrine, a condition that can cause a heart attack. We call this the "broken heart syndrome." I have seen it in action three times in the last five years. The arteries are perfect, the blood is flowing freely, and the mind is clear and filled with hope. Then the loss causes an extreme stress on the body. The resultant chemical changes precipitate a heart attack. When the spouse passes away, the remaining partner is much more likely to develop a health problem even if he or she was previously healthy. There is a change of chemistry when a source of love is lost. Some people are able to recover from the loss and rebuild their lives. Some cannot, and eventually, they actually die of broken hearts.

Which brings us back to my two dogs. If human love isn't readily available, pets can help improve a person's health. Those who allow an animal or two into their lives experience fewer heart attacks and infections and need fewer medications. People need love to recover from a loss of love. Nothing else is as powerful and long lasting.

The Opposite of Love

Love changes body chemistry for the good. Conversely, selfishness—the very opposite of love—can change body chemistry for the worse. Living a life centered on your own needs, your own desires, and your own specifications introduces dangerous chemical changes as well. Am I saying that a lack of love in this world is a determining factor in our present health crisis? Am I saying selfishness is just as destructive to the human mind, body, and spirit as eating low-fiber, high-fat, highly processed foods, living sedentary lifestyles, and filling our minds with the filth the media makes so readily available? Yes, that is *exactly* what I'm saying.

Selfishness is present in this world at many levels and is causing most, if not all, the stressors leading to disease. When Lucifer brought selfishness into God's perfect universe of love (remember that true love allows choices to be made), our present health care dilemma began. Selfishness was not a law that governed the universe. It was, in reality, an "antilaw." It generated stress, and this stress set in motion the negative chemical reactions with which we battle to this day. We were created to be with God, to live our lives encircled, supported, and sustained by His love. But Adam and Eve chose to turn their backs on God. They switched paths and began heading down the road that leads to eternal death. The bottom line? They chose to live separated from God, separated from the source of true love, and separated from the healing power that drives the universe. Human genetics became altered, body chemistry changed dramatically, chronic diseases developed, and death became everyone's ultimate destination. That is what happens when one lives apart from God. That is what happens when one lives outside of the powerful forces of life-sustaining love.

But it was that very force—the force of love—that handed a compass to a lost humanity. "God loved the world so much that he gave his one and only Son, so that everyone who believes in him will not perish but have eternal life" (John 3:16). God gave us the ultimate expression of love when He gave His Son.

"God showed how much he loved us by sending his one and only Son into the world so that we might have eternal life through him. This is real love—not that we loved God, but that he loved us and sent his Son as a sacrifice to take away our sins. Dear friends, since God loved us that much, we surely ought to love each other" (1 John 4:9-11).

Love is the solution to our global health care dilemma. Love opens the door for us to rediscover the ultimate prescription and find healing for our minds, bodies, and spirits. Love is the ultimate treatment. It's the final step to a full, long-lasting recovery.

Of course, the evil one wants to dupe us into thinking we can't find love on this earth, that we can't find happiness and fulfillment in a growing relationship with God. He whispers to us, *God doesn't love you! You must find other paths to healing. You must depend on certain sets of medications, specific doctrines, good deeds, the proper diet, giving your money to the poor, and living your life as others define it.* The lie first spoken in Eden—"You won't die!"—continues to echo in our minds and hearts today. And we are still taking the bait.

Now, however, you know better. You have discovered the ultimate prescription and are ready to introduce this amazingly powerful "medicine" into your life. When you do, you will experience—perhaps for the first time ever—the healing properties God placed within this divine law.

So get ready to continue your journey to optimum health. This final step will bring you a degree of healing you never dreamed possible!

18

ULTIMATE HEALING

ONE DAY A YOUNG WOMAN walked into a fabric shop and hurried to the counter. "Excuse me, sir," she said to the owner. "I'm looking for some noisy, rustling, white material."

The proprietor thought for a moment and then guided his customer across the room to where several bolts of cloth lay on a shelf. "How about these?" he asked.

Wordlessly the woman picked up the first bolt, unwound a few feet of the fabric, and shook it while listening carefully. She did the same for the next bolt, and the next. Finally she smiled. "This one," she announced. "This cloth is perfect."

As the owner was measuring out the fabric, curiosity got the best of him. "If I may be so bold," he said, "why do you want *noisy* material?"

The woman smiled shyly. "Well, sir, I'm making a wedding gown, and my fiancé is blind. When I walk down the aisle, I want him to know when I've arrived at the altar, so he won't be embarrassed."

What love! What tender regard! And what a perfect picture of how God sometimes operates in our lives. There are moments when He gets downright noisy in His attempts to reveal His love for us. Just ask the children of Israel standing at the foot of Mount Sinai. Just ask the Roman guards on Calvary at the moment of Jesus' death when the earth shook and rocks split apart. Just ask Saul on the road to Damascus staring up into a blinding light as God speaks to him. Sometimes love shouts!

But there are other times when God reveals His love to us in less dramatic ways—when He speaks in the "sound of a gentle whisper" that Elijah heard as he stood at the entrance of a cave in which he had been hiding (1 Kings 19:12). God never stops trying. Whether He thunders or whispers, He is always speaking to those who are willing to listen to His words of affection and guidance. I pray that you are listening now.

Two Paths, Two Futures

We have identified two very different paths of living that lead to two very different futures. One path is tied directly into Creation and the laws God set in place during that incredible week. The other path follows the father of lies—the devil—as he lures men and women away from a loving relationship with their heavenly Father. One path is all about health, good chemistry, and life. The other is all about sickness, bad chemistry, and death.

Here's the question each of us needs to ask ourselves: "How do I really know which path I'm on?"

The answer has to do with symptoms. As a cardiologist, I am very interested in the whole concept of symptoms because they reveal so much about the underlying disease from which my patients may be suffering. If I have a clear understanding of their symptoms, I can do a pretty good job of forming a diagnosis.

Chest pains? Possibly restricted blood flow to the heart.

Dizziness and fainting? There might not be enough oxygen reaching the brain. Shortness of breath? Numbness in the arm? Confusion? Slurred speech? All may be indications that something serious and unseen is taking place inside the body.

Those two paths—God's path and Satan's path—generate nonphysical "symptoms." On God's path—when we are living in harmony with His *spiritual* laws, laws governing the universe—we are more hopeful, confident, and accepting of others' faults. We find it easier to forgive and move on. On Satan's path, the spiritual picture is quite different. Our hearts fill with despair, anger, resentment, and unrelenting guilt. On this pathway, we live in fear of the very God who longs to save us from our sinful selves.

There is also a *physical* component to this journey. Only on God's path do we find true healing. Optimum health isn't dependent on a prescription drug or a miracle cure. It's not available over the counter or online. Optimum health comes when we live in harmony with God's health laws.

What are the physical symptoms of following Satan's path—of turning our backs on what God intended when He created us? They can include lifestyle-related conditions such as diabetes, heart disease, obesity, cancers, and shortened life spans. Even people who love God and enjoy a rich and rewarding relationship with their Creator can suffer greatly from these lifestyle diseases and end up in early graves if they refuse to follow God's Health Plan. They find themselves depending on modern medicine or giving in to the incredible pressure of appetite to form the foundation of their lives. When it comes to their physical health, they walk the wrong path and pay dearly for their choices. I see it all the time.

Conversely, some who come into my office follow Eden's ideal to the letter and yet still suffer from illness because they refuse to allow love, the Spirit of God, to rule their lives. They eat the right foods yet hate their neighbors. They exercise daily yet cheat on their taxes. They breathe in plenty of fresh air and drink ample amounts of pure water, yet they fill their minds with the senseless and violent content modern media makes so readily available.

Here's the point: our spiritual and physical lives cannot operate independently of each other. We cannot walk on both God's and Satan's path at the same time and expect good results. The interconnection between the mind and the body is so overpowering that trying to serve both masters brings only disaster.

This describes my patient David. He loved his family and attended church regularly, yet he strolled merrily along, following his own path when it came to his physical health. Obeying the Ten Commandments won't do a thing to help you physically if your eating habits are clogging your arteries. You can shut yourself up in a monastery and pray twenty-four hours a day, but you could die young of obesity-related diseases because you don't get any exercise. You simply cannot live your life with one foot on God's path and one foot on Satan's path and expect to enjoy optimum health. It's not going to happen. You have to place both feet firmly on God's path if you hope to live a healthy life. There is simply no other way.

So, where does the ultimate prescription come in? What part does love play in this incredible drama? The answer is simple—and beautiful. The ultimate prescription is what motivates and empowers us to change paths. It's where we discover love for the God who made us and find the strength to stop believing Satan's lies about Him. It's where we learn to love those we serve, even if some are unkind and ungenerous toward us. Most important, it's where we learn to love ourselves as children of God. People who are filled with this type of love would never knowingly do anything to harm others or themselves—and that includes breaking even one of God's health laws.

We Christians are often taught to concentrate on others more than ourselves. There is certainly wisdom in that. But there's a danger, too. To enjoy optimum health, we have to learn to love ourselves. We have to believe God when He tells us, through the apostle Paul, "Don't you realize that your body is the temple of the Holy Spirit, who lives in you and was given to you by God? You do not belong to yourself, for God bought you with a high price. So you must honor God with your body" (1 Corinthians 6:19-20).

Knowing this, what are you putting into your mind and body temple? Do your life and your body honor God? Do you have both feet firmly on the right path, or do you need to make some changes in your life? Are you on your way to experiencing ultimate healing?

A Matter of Worship

Probably the most profound question we need to ask ourselves when it comes to experiencing that longed-for ultimate healing is "Whom do we worship?"

Worship takes many forms—all of which affect our chemistry. Our worship may include attending a weekly church service, spending time out in nature, taking a walk, watching a sunset, listening to the ocean, smelling the fresh air, or seeing a smile. Worship might be helping a friend, offering a thankful prayer, singing a song, or writing a letter.

Now this may surprise you, but we actually become like what we worship—that is how profound the effect of worship is on our minds and bodies. If we spend time communing with God, we become more like Him, seeing life through His eyes, responding to situations as He would respond—all of which bring healing forces into our body. But if we bow at Satan's altar, if we worship other "things," we become selfish, angry, fearful—emotions that damage the body and can undo many of the good things we do for it.

But here's the most exciting part. As we worship God, we

begin to better understand the truth about this world and our place in it. We learn to avoid deception. We find we have the power to make the changes that those truths demand—the very truths I have tried to introduce to you in this book. We discover the proper place for modern medicine and for alternate ways of healing. We actually enjoy the process of exploring new avenues for bringing sound nutrition and intelligent exercise into our lives. We begin to change outwardly—and inwardly. Our chemistry adjusts to the new way of living, and we find that we feel better, sleep better, and experience a closer walk with God.

Then something absolutely miraculous happens. When we put the interests of others above our own, we become healers—people who bring healing hope to the minds and bodies of those around us. They, in turn, become healers to those within their circles of influence—the home, the church, the community. We all become "healing missionaries," and in the process, change the chemistry of countless people—everyone from the teenager behind the counter at the grocery store to the struggling neighbor who lives down the street. The love we share acts like a powerful medicine, easing heartaches and pain, motivating people to return to the source of ultimate healing. There is no drug, no medical procedure, no treatment that can accomplish this degree of restoration. The ultimate prescription acts like an energizing force in countless lives, transforming people in ways they never thought possible.

But don't expect your healing ministry to be easy or universally accepted. The ultimate prescription must be strong.

What Is Right?

I always enjoy my visits with Roland. A few years ago, he underwent successful surgery on his stenotic mitral valve. Since his surgery, he has continued to do well, is on a blood thinner to help lower the risk of stroke, and takes another medication to help control the speed of his atrial fibrillation—modern medicine at its best.

Over the years, Roland has made the slow adjustment to retirement. For a man who was in ministry in every corner of the world, being away from the front lines of evangelism has been quite a challenge.

Some time ago he came in for a physical and checked out just fine. During our conversation, I mentioned this book and how I felt the Spirit of God leading me to write about what some are thinking but few dare to say. I described the possible backlash I would experience because I was stepping on a lot of toes within my own profession. The "powers that be" would probably not be enthralled by a book that pointed to the "Great Physician" as the true source of all healing, and I shared my concern that the book might fail to reach those who needed it the most.

Roland thought for a moment and then told me this story.

Although he was in a very important leadership position when his grandson was born, he found himself wanting to spend as much time as possible with the little boy. Sometimes, because he was taking time to be part of his grandson's life, he would arrive late for meetings at work.

One day Roland walked into the busy day care center to pick up his grandson. The room was full of people and noise. The child, even though he was across the room, sensed the man's presence and, despite the chaos, moved toward his grandfather. Their eyes locked, and the little one cried out, "Papa!" with great love. This was the first time the little boy had ever spoken.

As Roland told me the story, I could see tears of joy in his eyes. Then he looked at me and said, "Jim, you have to do what is right, even if no one else in the world understands but you and God. The long-term rewards are always worth it when you put love for others first. People may not understand you, but in the end, following the Spirit's leading is the ultimate gratification."

I needed to hear that.

When we love others, when we make them laugh, when we help them along life's way, we are giving them a great prescription. We are changing their chemistry; we are flooding their systems with endorphins as we lower their levels of adrenaline and other harmful elements. We are helping to heal them. We are sharing the heart of love.

Roland related to me how he had worked with great healers all over the world. These were medical missionaries who served gladly, contented to grow in the places God had planted them. I decided then and there that I want to incorporate Roland's vision of service not only into my cardiology practice but also into my life. I want to be content in whatever place I am called to serve. I want to grow where God plants me. I want to help heal a diseased world. And more than that, someday I want to see my heavenly "Papa" and run into His arms, because I know He took the time and made the necessary sacrifices to teach me how to love.

The Long Journey

Many people come to my office just to ask questions because they have concerns. They may have worries about a leaky valve, a question about a medication, or the fear about an "unusual feeling" in their chest. When their concerns are met, when they learn the truth—no matter how simple or complex it may be— they feel reassured. This reassurance makes them feel better as the doubt that was creating a negative chemical environment deep inside them is replaced by the peace that comes from knowing the truth.

Our Great Physician is waiting to reassure us. He wants to

demonstrate His love and let us know that He is constantly available to help keep us on the right path—on His path. Most of all, He wants us to come to know true love, and this can occur only as we maintain a daily relationship with Him. This interaction with our Creator improves our chemistry and allows our doubts and fears to vanish. Peace floods our hearts, and health floods our bodies.

This amazing relationship was originally formed in the Garden of Eden as God revealed His love for Adam and Eve. The animals, the plants, the work that needed to be done, God's health laws—all were manifestations of this loving relationship. There were no doubts, no bad chemistry, no need for healing, no stress. Love ruled the day.

But then Adam and Eve opened the door to sin, and everything changed. They believed Satan's lies, and immediately selfishness and doubt entered their hearts. The perfect world began its long journey toward oblivion.

As time passed, dishonesty took root. Perceptions of God changed. The evil one constantly fed the world a diet of doubts and misconceptions—lies that have been passed down through the generations. Because God valued His lost relationship with His children, He provided laws to remind people of what love looked like. He called spokespeople to keep them on track. But few listened.

Finally He sent His Son to personally reconnect us with the only true source of ultimate healing. Even though we hung Him on the cross, the message of God's love remains.

Today we are in the targets of Satan's final trick—creating a false sense of security generated by our almost total dependence on modern medicine, high-tech science, and a belief that the answers we seek can be found in our own intelligence.

But God wants us to know the truth. He walks through the

garden of our lives calling us by name, inviting us to join Him on the path that leads to ultimate healing.

Right now, at this moment, wherever you are, answer the call. Ask the Holy Spirit to take control of not only your thoughts but also how you care for your body. Enter into a fresh, new, exciting, healing relationship with your heavenly Father. God says, "Look! I stand at the door and knock. If you hear my voice and open the door, I will come in, and we will share a meal together as friends" (Revelation 3:20).

The Creator wants to lead you back to the original plan He established at Creation. He is waiting to help you break away from Satan's lies and return to the one true God. He is waiting to walk with you on your journey to optimum health.

In the heavenly Father there is hope for the sickest person. There is hope for those who suffer with chronic pain. There is hope for incurable disease. There is hope for those who have chosen through the years to ignore how they were designed to live. This hope is found in a relationship with our Creator, who will bring us back to truth and reveal deception at every level of life. This relationship will bring us back to the ultimate prescription—to love, the governing force in the universe. No matter where you are on this journey, that relationship will be there with you, keeping you on the right path.

So come back to love. Choose to embrace and enjoy the eternal benefits found only through the ultimate prescription.

APPENDIX 1: SYMPTOMS

AT SOME POINT, many people have or will have problems with their hearts. Therefore, a basic explanation of what those problems look and feel like will enhance the understanding of the medical jargon they'll hear as they fight to regain health.

When part of a system is not functioning correctly, sooner or later problems develop. A car with a hole in its gas tank may run for a while, but eventually it will stop. Some vacuum cleaners will not work without a belt. A dishwasher without soap will have a problem cleaning dishes. Similarly, if the cardiovascular system is not working correctly, sooner or later problems will develop. Here is an example.

Mr. Gregory, fifty-two, was and still is an active man. But for six months he had been feeling something "different" inside. Lately, those feelings were coming on more frequently.

In the evening he walked his dog. There was a small hill in the middle of their route through the neighborhood. Every time Mr. Gregory walked up the hill, he felt a heavy sensation in his chest. He also experienced shortness of breath. Six months prior he could have made it up the hill without any problem, but now he stopped five or six times before reaching the top. Mr. Gregory was experiencing *mild to moderate* symptoms.

Symptoms are either feelings that are not normal for an individual, or they are a change in an individual's condition. Mr. Gregory eventually got help, but he took a chance by waiting.

Wayne O'Neal, a corporate lawyer, was at work early one morning. While preparing for a conference, he experienced severe chest pain. After collapsing, he was rushed to the emergency department of a local hospital. Mr. O'Neal was experiencing *severe* symptoms.

Unfortunately, many of us wait too long to find help when something "isn't right." The cardiovascular system is wonderfully made, but nothing is perfect. The system can break down under certain circumstances. How do we know when there's a problem? We hope that a *symptom* will be our first clue. Mr. O'Neal had no choice but to get help.

Mr. Scott, sixty-five, had just retired and was planning a vacation to the Pacific Northwest. He was fairly active and did some farming; however, he had not felt well for two months. He was tired, couldn't catch his breath, and noticed his legs swelling.

His family tried to get him to see the doctor, but he had other, "more important," things to do.

One day while in the fields, he collapsed. By the time he arrived in the emergency department, his heart had stopped. The medical team could not help him.

My point is this: we must pay close attention to our bodies. When something is not right, we need to consider this a warning sign and seek help. And if you know others who are having problems, encourage them to seek help sooner rather than later. It's easier to deal with a small problem than with a catastrophe.

Individuals are unique; each person feels different when the cardiovascular system is not working well. Not every person with heart disease will have a symptom. People without obvious symptoms are the most difficult to help and evaluate. In fact, the people without symptoms are more likely to notice that they do not feel "normal." This may be their only symptom.

Now let's take a look at the more common symptoms that occur when the cardiovascular system malfunctions.

Chest Pain

Chest pain is a very common symptom of cardiovascular disease. It can come from many different sources, including the heart. One might not feel "classic" pain. But a discomfort or "funny feeling" in the chest, arms, jaw, neck, teeth, and even the back could be related to the heart. The discomfort might feel like squeezing or pressing. In my years as a cardiologist, I have heard pain described in many different ways, but always I hear people say, "Something isn't right."

Angina is used to describe a condition of discomfort caused by decreased blood flow to the heart. These abnormal feelings may mean the heart is not getting enough blood.

I once saw a gentleman who experienced angina in his back. Sometimes discomfort in the stomach indicates angina. Often patients think they have indigestion, when in reality their pain is related to the heart. Discomfort brought on consistently by exertion, strong emotions, or even a big meal is a particular concern.

Sometimes pain or discomfort lasts for long periods of time. In this case, an individual could be experiencing a heart attack. A heart attack occurs when the blood flow supplying nourishment to the heart is cut off completely. Some say a heart attack feels like an elephant is sitting on their chests. But a heart attack can feel many different ways. The pain or discomfort might start in the front of the chest and move to the arm, neck, jaw, stomach, or back. There might be other feelings, including shortness of breath, weakness, dizziness, sickness of the stomach, sweating, an abnormal heartbeat, and/or clammy skin.

However, all prolonged chest pain is not necessarily a heart attack or angina. In fact, acid in the stomach, sprained chest muscles, problems with the lungs or esophagus, and other internal conditions can cause pain or discomfort in the upper body as well.

Nevertheless, when these symptoms appear, I want you to think that something might not be right with the heart. Call 911 and get help right away. Never drive yourself to the hospital; this would put you and others at great risk.

I want to reemphasize that chest pain can present itself in a variety of ways. I often hear excuses like these:

- It's just heartburn.
- I'm too young to have a heart problem.
- The pain isn't too bad—I'll just wait to see if it goes away.
- I don't think this is my heart.
- I'm too busy to get help.
- I don't want to be a bother to my family.
- It's the middle of the night—I'll wait until morning.
- No one in my family has had heart problems.

Don't make excuses. The sooner you get help, the better. *Do not* be embarrassed to ask for help. Doing so may save your life.

Other Symptoms

A Racing Heart

A racing heart might represent a problem. You might feel a fluttering, a skipping, a heavy pounding, or a jumpy feeling. Others may call these symptoms *palpitations.*

Dizziness, Light-Headedness, Passing Out

Though many conditions can cause these feelings, they can be associated with serious heart conditions. In particular, the electrical system may not be working well. It's imperative that the possible causes of these abnormal feelings be evaluated.

Collapse
This is a very serious problem. It warrants immediate medical attention because the cause could be life threatening.

Shortness of Breath
Dyspnea (pronounced **disp**-nee-uh) is the medical term for shortness of breath. This could represent a cardiovascular malfunction. Sometimes an individual unknowingly restricts activities because he or she cannot get a good breath. Typically it is difficult to sort out why an individual is short of breath because many different conditions can cause this feeling. For example, physical exertion in a nonactive person can cause dyspnea. But a prolonged period of dyspnea could be a sign of a more serious problem.

Swelling
The medical term for this symptom is *edema* (pronounced e-**dee**-ma). Fluid may collect in the legs, hands, or abdomen. At times, fluid collects in the lungs, which could cause shortness of breath.

Unusual Fatigue
Feeling tired much of the time may represent a medical problem and should be evaluated by a doctor.

Coughing
Prolonged coughing episodes or unexplained coughing associated with lying down needs to be evaluated. An adverse heart condition could be the cause.

Unable to Breathe Comfortably When Lying Flat
The medical term for this condition is *orthopnea* (pronounced orth-**op**-nee-uh). This could be related to the heart.

Skin Discoloration
If the skin has a bluish color, this could be a sign of inadequate blood flow and might indicate a heart malfunction.

Headache
I hear about this common symptom daily. A headache could be related to cardiovascular disease; the blood pressure might be elevated.

Other Symptoms
I want to emphasize that some groups of people—diabetics and the elderly, for example—may experience mild or unusual symptoms, making a heart problem more difficult to detect. Also, women often do not have the typical symptom of "chest pain."

If you're experiencing any of the symptoms mentioned, I hope you've already been evaluated by a doctor. The sooner a problem is analyzed, the better.

The following chart gives common symptoms related to the heart, the possible abnormality causing the symptom, and the general medical term describing the cardiac abnormality. The numerals in parentheses refer to the list of explanations following the chart.

Symptom	Possible Cardiovascular System Abnormality	General Medical Term (1)
Chest pain (2)	Complete blockage of a coronary artery leading to the heart	Myocardial infarction (heart attack)
	Partial blockage	Angina
	Opening and closing of a coronary artery	Coronary spasm
	Inflammation of the outside lining of the heart	Pericarditis (**pear**-i-card-**i**-tis)
	Abnormality of a heart valve	Mitral valve prolapse or Aortic stenosis
	Tear in the large artery leaving the heart (aorta)	Dissection
	Abnormal fast beating of the heart; an electrical system abnormality	Tachyarrhythmia (**tack**-ee-uh-**rhyth**-me-uh) (3)
Shortness of breath (dyspnea)	Complete blockage of a coronary artery	Myocardial infarction
	Partial blockage of a coronary artery	Angina
	Abnormality in the heart valves	Valvular heart disease, Mitral regurgitation, Mitral stenosis, Aortic regurgitation, Aortic stenosis
	Heart beating too slow or too fast	Bradyarrhythmia or Tachyarrhythmia (3)
	Weak heart muscle	Cardiomyopathy

Symptom	Possible Cardiovascular System Abnormality	General Medical Term (1)
Dizziness, loss of consciousness, or passing out (syncope)	Heart going too slow or too fast	Bradyarrhythmia (**brady**-uh-**rhyth**-me-uh) or Tachyarrhythmia
	Complete or partial blockage of a coronary artery	Myocardial infarction or angina
	Heart valve not opening	Aortic stenosis
	Artery blockage in neck vessel (brain does not get enough blood with oxygen)	Cerebral Vascular Accident (CVA) or stroke (4)
Swelling (edema)	Heart muscle weak (5)	Cardiomyopathy
Heart racing or palpitations	Abnormality in electrical system	Tachyarrhythmia (3)
Unusual fatigue (6)	Weak heart	Cardiomyopathy
	Abnormal electrical system (heart going too slow or too fast)	Bradyarrhythmia or Tachyarrhythmia (3)
Coughing (7)	Fluid building up in the lungs	Pulmonary edema
Unable to breathe comfortably when lying down (orthopnea)	Fluid building up in the lungs (8)	Pulmonary edema
Headache (9)	High blood pressure in the arteries	Hypertension (10)
Skin discoloration (11)	Insufficient oxygenated blood in the body	

1. The abnormalities listed have been limited to the more common malfunctions of the cardiovascular system. The origin of the abnormality has not been specified.
2. There are many causes of chest pain that are unrelated to the cardiovascular system, but it is beyond the scope of this book to list them all.
3. There are many different types of fast heart rates (*tachyarrhythmias*) and slow heart rates (*bradyarrhythmias*).
4. More discussion of this later.
5. There are numerous reasons why a heart muscle can be weak. For more information, see the references to weakened hearts in appendixes 2 and 3.
6. There are many other causes of fatigue unrelated to the cardiovascular system.
7. There are many other noncardiac causes of a cough, from a simple cold to sinus drainage.
8. There could also be other causes.
9. Headache has many other noncardiovascular causes.
10. Hypertension (high blood pressure) typically has no symptoms.
11. There are numerous causes of skin discoloration, including the heart's not pumping blood to the body, or wrong connections in the cardiovascular system. This is usually an abnormality occurring at birth (*congenital*) and is often detected at an early age.

When you discover a symptom, you may need an evaluation, which can include diagnostic testing. There are many ways to evaluate symptoms. Unfortunately, sometimes doing so is not an easy task. It's important to see a doctor or other health care provider who can help.

APPENDIX 2: DIAGNOSTIC TESTING

Tom Gentry, forty-six, is a hardworking mechanic. Most people say he's the best in town. Tom had seen a physician about ten months before coming to my office. Tom wasn't a talkative person, but I could tell he would not have been seeing me unless something was wrong.

During the course of our conversation he told me that another doctor had wanted to "put me through the mill." Tom had decided he would rather risk dying than "be tortured by tests." I spent a long time convincing him that none of our testing was torture. Some tests might be a little uncomfortable, but knowing the cause of his symptoms would, in my opinion, be worth the risk of the testing. After that Tom said, "Couldn't I just have a pill to make me all better?"

I wish it were that simple. I explained to him that testing would help me know the cause of the problem. Once we identified the cause, we could give the right treatment. This might include medications, surgery, or factors in his lifestyle that needed to change.

To make a long story short, Tom had several tests. I was careful to explain why each was performed and what to expect during the routines. I also explained the risks. Having that knowledge seemed to help my patient tremendously. Understanding the tests decreased some of his fears and gave him confidence and a feeling of being in control. Eventually, Tom underwent heart surgery. This, along with some important lifestyle changes, returned my patient to a normal and productive life.

There are many methods your health care provider can use to evaluate your symptoms for heart disease. Below are brief descriptions of a few of the most common diagnostic testing procedures.

Evaluation Process

The evaluation process begins with words. A good health care provider will listen to you and talk with you first. Ideally you can describe in detail what makes you feel "not right." More questions might follow. This discussion can provide more information than the most advanced tests. The provider will ask questions regarding past medical problems and treatments. Having an up-to-date health record is important for both you and the provider in helping to understand the entire picture. If you're seeing a new provider, please bring your old records. It will expedite your care.

The Physical Examination

When the interview phase is completed, the provider is thinking, *What could be causing this feeling?* The next step will be a physical examination to give the provider more information. I consider the interview and the physical exam the most important parts in making a correct *diagnosis* (the medical term explaining the symptoms). During the physical exam the provider will observe you and your body and take your vital signs. Measuring the vital signs consists of feeling or listening to how fast your heart is going per minute, counting how many times you breathe in a minute, measuring the body temperature and blood pressure. The provider obtains your blood pressure by listening for sounds in your blood vessels while using a cuff device to squeeze your upper arm. This will measure the pressure in the cardiovascular system. This test is slightly uncomfortable because the cuff squeezes the arm, but it is certainly not unbearable.

Next the provider will examine and listen to your body. Skilled examiners are efficient, so this does not take too long, and there are really no risks or discomforts. The physical exam gives even more clues about the cause of your symptoms. Sometimes a cause will be found right away, and no further tests will be needed.

Further Tests

After talking to you and examining your body, the health care provider will decide whether further tests are needed and, if so, what specific tests would be most beneficial.

Following is an explanation of the most common tests used to evaluate the cardiovascular system.

Electrocardiogram (EKG or ECG)

This is a recording of the heart's electrical impulses. The test gives much information, including the rhythm of the heart, evidence of a heart attack, and thickening of the heart muscle. It could also aid in determining whether the heart is getting enough blood.

The test lasts about five minutes and is performed by placing small adhesive patches at specific locations on the chest, arms, and legs. These small patches are called electrodes. Usually the patient is lying down during the test, and the data from the test is recorded on special paper.

If a patient's chest is especially hairy, some of the hair may need to be shaved so that the electrodes have better contact with the skin. This test has no significant risks or dangers. Rarely, there might be a slight skin reaction when the chest hair is shaved before the electrodes are placed.

Blood Work

A provider will ask for blood to be drawn, usually from the arm, and sent to the lab for analysis. Blood analysis gives information about the function of many of the internal organs. Troponin and creatinine phosphokinase (CPK) are common blood tests that help determine whether a heart muscle is dying or not getting enough nourishment.

Usually the cholesterol level is measured. For this test, the patient should have gone without food for twelve hours before the blood is drawn. *Atrial natriuretic peptide* is another blood test used to evaluate whether the heart is working efficiently.

To draw blood, a technician usually places a tourniquet on the arm above a vein. The test time is less than a minute if a vein is easily found. The entire area is cleaned to help prevent infection. A needle is inserted into the vein, and the blood is collected in a clean tube. There is a very small chance of bleeding, and some pain occurs (this varies from person to person) when the needle breaks the skin.

Sometimes a small sterile plastic device is placed into a vein and taped in place. This is called an IV (intravenous) procedure. This device is usually inserted into a vein in the arm or on the wrist. The tubing attached to the IV device allows fluids and medications to be given directly into the bloodstream for immediate action.

Echocardiography

An echocardiogram bounces sound waves off the various structures of the heart and constructs a picture. The moving picture gives a wealth of information that includes the structure and strength of the patient's heart, as well as the blood flow within the heart. The test might reveal if there has been a previous heart attack. This test also evaluates the heart valves.

First, two or three electrodes are placed on the chest to monitor the heart rhythm. A small device called a *transducer* is placed at different locations on the chest wall. Sound waves are sent from this device and bounce back, thus creating the picture. The patient usually lies on his or her left side on a special bed that has an area cut out so the transducer can be easily manipulated, but the patient is covered for privacy.

The sonographer (the person who obtains the pictures) will place the transducer, along with some gel, on the chest wall. The gel aids in obtaining the best pictures. The sonographer will change the position of the transducer many times during the test to look at the heart from a variety of angles. The images are permanently recorded on videotape or disc.

Sometimes the pushing feels uncomfortable. Some describe a tickling feeling. There's no preparation needed, and there are no significant risks to this test.

Holter Monitor

This test records every beat of the heart for twenty-four to forty-eight hours and helps to determine whether the heart's electrical system is malfunctioning. For example, the monitor will detect whether the heart is going too fast or too slow, skipping a beat, or even stopping briefly. The patient is asked to write in a diary the specific times he or she feels differently and the way he or she is feeling at those times. The health care provider can correlate symptoms with the heart's electrical system.

The patient wears a small monitoring device, usually placed on a belt around the waist. The device records the action of the heart and is attached to electrodes placed in a similar manner as in an EKG.

No specific preparation is needed. The risks are minimal to none.

Event Monitor

There are times when a patient has only occasional symptoms. The *event monitor* can record the heart's rhythm up to a month at a time. It's a device similar to the Holter monitor in terms of its placement on the body. When a symptom occurs, the patient activates the device, and the heart rhythm is recorded for a short period. The information is usually sent immediately to the health care provider. The patient is also given a diary to use during the testing period.

I once had a patient with very infrequent symptoms. I could not "catch" the symptoms on a Holter or event monitor. Today there are small devices that can be implanted below the skin in the chest wall to record every single heartbeat for as long as a year. I recommended using this device for my patient, and sure enough, in a few months, he felt symptoms. We discovered the type of electrical malfunction he suffered, which was easily treatable. Although these devices are rarely used, they are available.

Exercise Stress Test

In this test the patient is asked to place stress on the heart, usually by exercising. The provider monitors changes in the cardiovascular system by using a continuous EKG, checking the blood pressure frequently, and evaluating symptoms and exercise ability during the stress.

An exercise stress test gives information on whether there is adequate blood flow to the heart during conditions when the heart is working harder than usual. This test can also estimate the patient's level of cardiovascular fitness.

If the patient is able to walk, an exercise stress is used. The patient walks on a treadmill that increases in speed and incline over a period of time. A stationary bicycle can also be used in some situations. Exercise increases the heart rate. The provider monitors the EKG and asks frequently whether the patient is aware of any symptoms as the test proceeds. Blood pressure is measured often.

The stress test requires patients to go without food before the test, to wear comfortable walking clothes and shoes, and to be able to walk or pedal at increasing speeds. The risks are small. The main risk is developing symptoms while walking. I tell my patients, "I would rather have you develop a symptom when I was watching and could do something about it than have you develop symptoms at home." A minor skin irritation could also occur as the result of the electrode placement.

Some patients are unable to walk adequately on a treadmill. In this case, there are other types of nonexercise stress tests.

Stress Echocardiogram

In addition to the information obtained from a regular stress test, a stress echocardiogram gives pictures of the heart before and after exercise. The provider looks to see if the heart muscle performs differently after exercise. This added information provides another tool for detecting problems.

The test begins with an echocardiogram, described previously. The patient then walks on a treadmill. After the walk, while the heart is still beating fast, another set of pictures of the heart is obtained. These images, in addition to the information gained during the regular stress test, are reviewed to detect abnormalities. The risks and preparation for the test are as described for the stress test and the echocardiogram.

Nuclear Medicine Stress Test

A nuclear medicine stress test adds a different element to the normal stress test and enhances diagnostic abilities. As with the other stress tests, the provider is evaluating the blood flow to the heart muscle.

In addition to the stress test, a radioactive material (thallium or Cardiolite) is injected into a vein. The radioactive tracer travels throughout the heart and helps to evaluate blood flow.

The test is usually done in two stages. First, the patient lies flat and an X-ray machine takes pictures at various angles to get images of blood flow to the heart.

Next, the patient exercises. Again, a radioactive tracer is injected, and more images are obtained after the exercise. The provider then compares blood flow before the exercise with blood flow after the exercise. The comparison assists in detection of possible problems.

In preparation, the provider will ask you not to eat food for at least six hours before the test. You must also abstain from caffeine for forty-eight hours before the test. This is hard for some people because caffeine is in many of the items they eat and drink. The provider may ask you to hold off on taking certain medications, especially if these medications would affect the speed of your heart or your ability to exercise. Diabetics will receive special instructions regarding their blood-sugar medications. As with the regular stress test, casual clothes are recommended, along with shoes appropriate for walking. The entire test lasts about three hours.

The risks are similar to those for a regular stress test but with the added minimal risk of starting an IV and the rare chance of an adverse reaction to the radioactive material. There is also a very small risk of exposure to radiation, but the amount of radiation exposure is actually less than you would receive from having a regular chest X-ray.

Gated Scanning

Sometimes a nuclear stress test includes gated scanning. This test helps determine the overall strength, or pumping ability, of the heart. This scan is frequently used to evaluate whether medications—especially medications used to fight cancer—are weakening the heart muscle.

The test involves placing a radioactive tracer in the blood via an IV line that circulates to the heart. A nuclear camera then takes pictures that help evaluate the heart's pumping ability. The risks and preparation are similar to those for the nuclear stress test.

Nonexercise Stress Tests

When a patient is unable to walk on a treadmill, another type of stress to the heart might be needed. These tests involve use of medications (dobutamine) that speed up the heart or medications (adenosine or Persantine, to name just two) that cause the coronary arteries to become bigger. These agents are injected into a vein, and the examination evaluates blood flow to the heart before and after the stress that these medications provide. The EKG, blood pressure, and symptoms are monitored continually during the testing.

Before the medication is injected into a vein, X-ray images of the heart are made—the same as for a regular nuclear examination. The patient is lying down for the procedure and is under constant monitoring while the medication is injected. Another set of X-ray pictures of the heart is taken fifteen to thirty minutes later. The sets of pictures are compared to evaluate whether the heart is getting sufficient blood. The images are stored on computer discs for future reference.

The risks are small and include those of the regular nuclear test. There is also the risk of an adverse reaction to the medication given to stress the heart. Again, the risks are small compared to the benefit of a diagnosis. The preparation is usually the same as for the nuclear test. Your provider will guide you as to which medications to take or avoid before the test.

Transesophageal Echocardiogram (TEE)

In this examination, a small device called a *probe* is passed into the esophagus. The *esophagus* is a tube located behind your heart that takes food from your mouth to your stomach. From the vantage point of the esophagus, the device can obtain clear pictures of the heart. The information gained is similar to that offered by an echocardiogram. The TEE is used when clear pictures of the heart cannot be obtained from the transthoracic (chest) views.

Sometimes this test is used when a patient has suffered an injury to the chest wall or has an extremely large chest. This test can also give specific information on valvular structure and function, because it can also visualize parts of the heart that a regular echocardiogram cannot evaluate well.

During this examination, two or three electrodes, placed on the chest, continuously monitor the rhythm of the heart. An IV, usually placed into a vein in the arm or wrist area and attached to tubing, allows fluid and medications to be given directly into the bloodstream for immediate action. An *oximeter*—a small device placed on the finger—monitors the oxygen level in the body. Supplemental oxygen is usually given to keep the blood oxygen level high during the test. The gag reflex is usually suppressed with a spray numbing the back of the throat.

Medication is used to relax the patient, but he or she may feel the tube as it is passed through the throat. The flexible tube is gently passed through the mouth and into the esophagus while the patient lies on his or her left side. Once the probe is in place, the images of the heart are recorded. The exam usually lasts about fifteen to twenty minutes, depending on how much information is needed. You might ask, "If the pictures are so clear, why not perform this test on everyone?" The test is more uncomfortable than others and has a few more risks. No one likes to have a probe passed into his or her esophagus.

There are also more risks for the TEE than for a regular echo-cardiogram. The main risk comes from the IV medications given: an adverse reaction or side effect could occur. Also, any time an IV is started, there can be a small risk of bleeding. When the probe is passed into the esophagus, there is a minimal chance of damage to the teeth or the back of the throat. Close monitoring is required to minimize these risks. The test is usually performed in a hospital because of the need for the monitoring devices and possible risks, but the patient usually goes home the same day. The patient might have a sore throat after the procedure. The patient should wait to eat until the throat is no longer numb.

In preparation for the test, patients must have an empty stomach, because there is a risk of vomiting during the test. If patients are on a daily medication, the provider may have them take their medication at least two hours before the procedure. Because of the risks involved, the provider gives a very detailed explanation to the patient. The provider will ask patients to sign a consent form, which states that they have received an explanation of the procedure and understand the test and the risks involved. As you can see, the risks are not too great, but they are present. The provider should take every precaution to minimize the risks and to ensure patients understand them before the exam.

Heart Catheterization (Coronary Angiography)

In a *cardiac catheterization* a small plastic tube called a *catheter* is positioned at various locations within the heart. The information acquired includes visualization of the coronary arteries and any blockages that might be present, the strength of the heart, and measurements of pressure within the heart. The procedure lasts from thirty to sixty minutes. This test gives the cardiologist a great deal of information and often provides definitive answers regarding cardiovascular system abnormalities. For instance, if a stress test is abnormal, heart catheterization can verify the results of the stress test and gauge the severity of the problem. The procedure determines the nature of blockages in the arteries, which indicates to the cardiologist the best treatment to recommend. The information regarding the strength of the heart and the pressures within the heart chambers is also very useful.

In preparation, the provider explains the risk and benefits of the procedure—just as I am doing now—and asks the patient to sign a consent form. The patient has blood drawn to make sure blood counts are good, the kidneys are functioning well, and there are no clotting abnormalities. An EKG and a chest X-ray are usually performed to provide baseline data. If diabetes, kidney disease, hypertension, or other adverse medical conditions are present, the provider may give specific instructions. The patient will be advised concerning which medications to take before the test. The provider also completes a written medical history of the patient before the test to give that information to those who may need it.

Ideally, the stomach is empty before the procedure. If the test is scheduled as an outpatient procedure, I ask patients not to eat anything after midnight. They can have sips of water to take their regular medications. Sometimes an adjustment on diabetic medications needs to be made. Patients must have someone drive them home after the procedure.

The actual procedure is performed in the hospital or a special outpatient center. If the patient is not already in the hospital, an IV will be started upon arrival in the holding area. The patient should also go to the bathroom before entering the catheterization suite. Sometimes women will also have a urinary catheter inserted into the bladder. If the patient is to be given relaxing medications, those will usually be given at this point. The provider reviews the patient's charts to make sure all preliminary preparation has been completed. The catheterization suite is the room where the procedure is done. The patient will be positioned on a table that is surrounded by an X-ray camera, which will move to various locations during the procedure to take the pictures from many different angles. There will be several monitors, usually on the left side of the patient. This enables the cardiologist to visualize the heart, observe pressures within the cardiovascular system, and monitor the heart rhythm. The patient might also see a control room where technicians assist with the procedure.

After the patient has been positioned on the table, electrodes are placed on the chest to monitor the heart rhythm. The area over the right and left groin will be cleaned and shaved. A drape will be placed over the entire body. This will help keep the procedure clean (sterile). The technician will hook up the needed equipment. At this point, if the patient has not been given a medication by mouth to help him or her relax, it will be administered by IV. The patient will be awake during the catheterization, as the medical team will need to be able to communicate with him or her.

Injecting a medication called Xylocaine with a small needle will numb the area over the entry site for the catheter, usually the right groin. Depending on the circumstances, other entry sites are sometimes needed. The injection of the numbing medication feels like a large bee sting. The cardiologist will give numbing medication over the entire area. At this point the patient should start feeling relaxed and should feel no significant discomfort. The cardiologist then places a small device called a *sheath* into an artery. The sheath is used to carefully pass catheters (long, thin, plastic tubes) through the artery and into or near the heart. This allows the cardiologist to gather the needed data. The patient does not feel the passing of the catheters. The cardiologist is able to see where the catheters are going by looking at a monitor.

Special contrast material (dye) is injected into the coronary arteries and X-ray pictures are taken. The contrast material makes the arteries of the heart visible on the X-rays, and the images taken are recorded for future review. The strength of the heart is measured by placing contrast material into the left ventricle, and pictures are taken as the heart pumps. There may be a very warm sensation, or "hot flash," as the contrast agent is pumped throughout the body. If needed, the test can also measure pressures in various parts of the cardiovascular system.

After the diagnostic procedure, the patient will go to a recovery area. If no additional treatment is needed during recovery, the sheath will be removed. Some cardiologists apply direct pressure over the entry site for about twenty minutes, until any bleeding stops. Other cardiologists use a special device inserted into the artery to seal the hole created by the sheath. In this case, direct pressure is not needed. The patient will need to remain fairly still, lying on his or her back for several hours after the procedure. If the patient needs to use the bathroom, a urinal will be provided.

While the patient is in a supine position (lying on the back), the provider will monitor the patient closely to check for bleeding. If there are no complications, the patient may eat but must still continue to lie fairly flat. After a period of time determined by the cardiologist, the patient will be able to move around and go home, pending the results of the test. Once home, the patient should be careful to limit physical activities. The cardiologist will give specific discharge instructions.

A heart *catheterization* is termed an *invasive procedure* because the catheter is considered to be "invading" the body. There are definitely more risks than in the previous tests described in this appendix. The risks include, but are not limited to, the following:

- Adverse reaction to the medication given for relaxation
- Bleeding at the entry site
- Damage to the blood vessels from the sheath and catheters
- Damage to the kidney from the contrast material
- Heart attack
- Stroke
- Adverse reaction to the contrast material
- Abnormal heart rhythms

Although the risk of serious complications is very small, there is also even a small risk of death. I would not recommend this test unless the benefits of knowing what is causing the symptoms outweigh the risks.

Electrophysiologic Testing (EP Testing)

I need to briefly mention a sophisticated form of testing of the electrical system. EP testing allows the cardiologist to determine whether the electrical system of the heart is malfunctioning and, if so, to identify the specific causes of the malfunction. This test might determine whether the electrical system firing is too slow, too fast, or irregular.

A specialized cardiologist, called an electrophysiologist, performs this test in a laboratory very much like a catheterization suite. The procedure is similar to the heart catheterization already described, in that sheaths are placed in a vein or an artery in the groin area and catheters are passed through them. However, in this procedure, specialized catheters are passed through the sheaths into exact locations in the heart to obtain information on the electrical system.

This test is recommended for any of the following symptoms:

- When an individual has had a cardiac collapse relating to the electrical system
- If previous testing has demonstrated certain types of dangerous rhythm patterns not managed with medications
- If further information relating to the electrical system is needed
- When a heart has been declared very weak

In some situations, the electrophysiologist can use energy to destroy certain electrical cells of the heart that are causing the abnormal rhythms. This is called an *ablation*. At other times the specialist can implant small devices that monitor the heart and restore normal rhythms should an abnormality develop. These devices are called automatic internal cardiac defibrillators.

This test takes longer than a regular catheterization, but the preparation is similar. However, in addition to the risks mentioned for a regular heart catheterization, there is also the increased risk of causing a dangerous heart rhythm. Again, this test would not be done if the benefits of testing did not outweigh the risks.

More Sophisticated Tests

The last few years have seen the development of a number of even more sophisticated tests to evaluate the heart. These tests are growing in use and availability. The following is a list of these noninvasive tests, along with a brief description of each one.

Multisliced Computerized Tomography
(CT Scan of the Heart)

This test uses X-rays and computerized processing to make pictures of the heart and other blood vessels in the body. There are new advanced scanners, called *Ultrafast CT Scanners*, which can visualize the coronary arteries. This may lead to early detection of coronary artery disease. The risks of this procedure are minimal, and the benefits are currently being evaluated. This test may be able to replace the need for heart catheterization in many instances.

Magnetic Resonance Imaging (MRI)

This type of advanced test uses a magnetic field rather than X-rays to make images. Most MRIs use a moving platform in a circular tunnel and are quite noisy. Some people feel claustrophobic in these machines, although in recent years, new circular open MRIs have been developed, which minimize that problem. The MRI gives detailed information on the heart structures. This test is used infrequently.

Carotid Ultrasound

This common test uses sound-wave energy to provide information about the large arteries of the neck—specifically blockages in these arteries. Ultrasound can also look at the large artery in the abdomen—the aorta—as well as the arteries of the legs to evaluate for abnormalities.

Echocardiogram with Contrast Agents

Sometimes special agents are given through an IV while an echocardiogram is being performed. Contrast agents are used when a regular echocardiogram does not show the heart structures well. These agents enable the cardiologist to better visualize the heart structures. The preparation is the same as a regular echocardiogram. There is a small risk of adverse reaction to the contrast agent.

Positron-Emission Tomography

Sometimes called a *PET scan*, this test provides detailed information about blood flow to the heart. Radioactive material is given through an IV, and a sequence of images is recorded. The machine rotates around the body to capture many images. The patient will be in a supine position (on the back) in a device that looks like a large donut. PET scanning is very expensive and has limited availability. This test is rarely used in the evaluation of the heart.

Myths about Cardiac Testing

1. A negative stress test means I cannot have a heart attack. This is not true. A stress test may be positive if significant blockages are present in the coronary arteries. However, there is a chance that a significant blockage (or blockages) will not be picked up by a stress test. Currently, there is not a test that can predict who will have a heart attack. Maybe someday we will have such a test. In the meantime, risk factors help us identify persons who are more likely to have a heart attack.

2. If an EKG is normal, my heart is fine. This may or may not be true. You could be having a heart attack with a normal EKG.

This concludes an overview of the most common—but not all—diagnostic tests of the cardiovascular system. Keep in mind that if you have specific questions regarding any test ordered, you should ask your health care provider.

APPENDIX 3: TREATMENT

ONCE A DIAGNOSIS is made, the provider creates an individualized treatment plan. This plan should keep in mind a person's needs and preferences. There are many "right" treatments, but it is beyond the scope of this appendix to list every treatment for every condition. Here we will mention just some helpful, general principles.

Remember, knowledge is power. The more you know, the more you will be able to participate in your own care. We'll discuss the more common medical responses, beginning with acute treatment. *Acute treatment* is what must be done immediately.

Coronary Artery Disease (CAD)

Blockage in the arteries supplying the heart with blood is termed *coronary artery disease* (CAD) or *coronary arteriosclerosis*. We've already discussed symptoms and tests that represent and confirm CAD. CAD is the most common problem leading to a malfunction in the cardiovascular system. I'm going to explain CAD in a little more detail because a better understanding will help you learn about the treatment.

Every minute someone dies from CAD. It's the leading cause

of death in every community in America. It is also a growing problem worldwide. The problem develops because the coronary arteries become narrowed or blocked completely. When this occurs, blood with oxygen (nourishment) cannot reach the heart muscle. Typically, symptoms follow.

What causes the arteries to narrow? The body carries fats, called *lipids*, in the blood. Lipids can gradually build up inside the blood vessels. These buildups can become hardened, or *calcified*. Other elements become involved as well, making the blockages bigger and bigger. Blood has a hard time passing through the arteries and cannot reach its destination. When the heart muscle does not receive enough blood, symptoms develop. We discussed these symptoms in appendix 1.

Before we go further, I want to make a few points. The blockages in the arteries of the heart can also occur elsewhere in the body, including the arteries supplying the brain, legs, and other vital organs.

Sometimes a blockage—also called *plaque*—may become unstable. If this plaque, which you could think of as an artery "pimple," pops, there could be big problems, even if there is just a 30 to 40 percent narrowing in the artery.

When the "pimple" pops (ruptures), the body sees the rupture as an injury. If you had a cut on your arm, other cells would be recruited to fight the damage. Inside the arteries, cells are recruited to help fight the damage when a plaque ruptures. These cells mean well, but as they congregate around the rupture, they can clog the artery and lead to a heart attack.

Mr. Adams is a forty-year-old who had never had a medical problem in his life. One morning while getting ready for his job at the electric company, he developed excruciating chest pain. Testing revealed that a 30 percent plaque obstruction inside a coronary artery had ruptured, causing a heart attack.

Unfortunately, there are no diagnostic tests to predict which plaques will rupture. When Mr. Adams's plaque ruptured, the recruited damage-fighting cells formed a clot that resulted in a loss of blood flow in the artery. Severe pain resulted.

Mr. Adams's problem was diagnosed quickly, and treatment was begun. The cornerstone in the treatment of *acute* CAD is to first restore blood flow to the heart and then help prevent the development of further problems related to the lack of blood flow. *Chronic* treatment involves trying to halt or even reverse the disease process. This is called *regression* and is usually accomplished through diet and other lifestyle changes.

If blood flow is not restored quickly by opening the blocked artery, a heart attack will occur. This could lead to many serious problems. Because of the lack of blood flow to the heart, the electrical system could be damaged, resulting in the development of dangerous fast or slow heart rhythms. When these rhythms occur, the heart might be beating so rapidly or slowly that it is unable to pump blood throughout the body. In a heart attack, the heart muscle itself does not pump well because of an insufficient supply of oxygenated blood. Without oxygenated blood supplied by the heart, the other organs of the body cannot function.

The heart valves controlling the direction of blood flow depend on muscles that may be damaged during a heart attack. Blood flow might move in the wrong direction because the valve is not working properly. This is another major acute problem.

During a heart attack, it is even possible that a dead heart muscle may break open or rupture. This event is usually fatal. As you can see, getting immediate treatment could save your life.

If you think you're having a heart attack, sit down, call 911, and leave the phone off the hook so your call can be traced if you pass out. Take a blood-thinning aspirin if possible. Try your best to relax. Do not drive yourself to the hospital. If someone other than the paramedics takes you to the hospital (not the ideal), let everyone know immediately upon arrival that you think you are having a heart attack. This is not the time to be patient and wait your turn.

The acute treatment for a heart attack will focus on restoring blood flow to the part of the heart not getting blood, as well as treating the resulting problems previously mentioned if they occur. You will receive aspirin and oxygen. Often an emergency catheterization will be performed. This will help providers to decide whether you need a procedure called *angioplasty* to open the artery. This might be the first treatment option initiated, depending on the situation and availability. Sometimes clot-busting medications (*thrombolytics*) will be given through an IV to help open the artery. Depending on your condition, other medications to help the heart and prevent blood clots will be given as well.

Angioplasty (PTCA) uses the technique of heart catheterization. A catheter is inserted through an access point in an artery (usually in the groin) and is passed to the origin of the coronary arteries. Pictures of the arteries are obtained. In addition, a guiding catheter is passed to the blocked coronary artery.

Next, a second catheter with a balloon near the tip of the catheter is threaded through the guiding catheter. Once the balloon has reached the blockage, it is inflated to squish the blockage against the artery wall and restore blood flow. The balloon may be inflated several times. A small metal device called a *stent* is usually placed (deployed) in the artery to help keep it open. These devices, which look like a spring and are made of stainless steel, are designed to hold the artery open and help prevent further narrowing of the vessel, or restenosis.

The procedure has more risks than a heart catheterization.

The cardiologist performing the procedure will explain the risks. Drug-coated stents, along with medications to help prevent clotting, have greatly decreased the amount of restenosis and have enhanced the treatment of acute myocardial infarction. During and after the procedure, strong medications are administered to help prevent clotting and keep the blood "thin."

In addition to angioplasty and stents, there are other procedures currently in use to open arteries. *Atherectomy* is a process that uses a special device to remove the fatty plaque in the artery. This is sometimes called a "roto rooter" procedure. The plaque is scraped away using a special catheter. The plaque is either pulled out of the body or ground into very small particles and carried away by the bloodstream. Lasers are used infrequently to help open the coronary arteries.

Angioplasty and stenting are the most common procedures used to open arteries. However, these procedures do not remove the chance of a heart attack; they do allow more blood flow through the coronary artery, which helps the heart get more oxygen so that serious problems previously mentioned may be averted.

Bypass surgery (more on this later) is sometimes needed if angioplasty is not successful or if severe complications result from the heart attack. If the heart has an abnormally fast rhythm, it will need to be shocked (defibrillated) to restore a normal rhythm. If, during the heart attack, the heart is going abnormally slow, a device called a *pacemaker* will help speed up the heart. Medication is also given to help stabilize the abnormal rhythms.

After the initial event, the patient will be admitted to the hospital for several days for an uncomplicated heart attack. If there are complications, the hospital stay will be longer. The medical team will begin medications to restore optimal heart function. Preventive measures will be initiated. Finally, the patient's activity level will gradually be increased, and cardiac rehabilitation will begin.

Only about one-fourth of the people who could benefit from a rehabilitation program actually participate in such treatment. Rehab programs help all patients with heart disease and are a very important part of the treatment plan. The program serves to educate patients concerning the cardiac condition—to counsel, support, and teach preventative measures. In addition, the patient's physical activity will be gradually increased under a monitored situation. I cannot overemphasize the importance of a rehab program in an acute treatment plan.

Diagnostic testing might reveal that one or more of a patient's arteries are partially blocked and that a heart attack is looming in the future. In this case, the provider will create a specific individualized treatment plan. For instance, if blockages are not too severe, medications will be given to diminish the demands on the heart, along with aspirin and a cholesterol-lowering medication. If medications, preventive measures, and lifestyle changes are ineffective in controlling symptoms, the cardiologist may recommend a more invasive form of treatment. In situations of severe blockages in the arteries, the provider recommends an angioplasty or bypass surgery.

Sometimes medical therapy alone cannot control symptoms. If there are severe blockages in multiple coronary arteries or if the main branch of the coronary system is blocked, the cardiologist will recommend bypass surgery. It's important to note that some arteries are so severely diseased or so small that neither bypass surgery nor angioplasty would be beneficial. Heart catheterization provides this information to the health care provider.

Coronary Artery Bypass Surgery (CABS)

In the last twenty-five years, coronary artery bypass surgery (CABS) has become a common treatment for diseased arteries.

CABS involves taking an artery from the chest wall, or sections of veins from the legs, and attaching them to coronary arteries below the severe blockages, giving more blood flow to the heart. The transplanted bit of artery or vein is termed a *graft*. In some situations, arteries may be taken from the arm.

An artery tends to have fewer problems over time than veins from the leg, which are accustomed to lower pressures. Arteries have stronger walls, too. This new connection brings a new blood supply to the heart. Removal of the conduit (section of vein or artery from the source site) will not usually significantly affect blood flow in an individual's body.

A specialized surgeon, a cardiothoracic surgeon, performs the operation. The patient receives a general anesthetic, which will put him or her to sleep. For the surgery, different techniques are available. Traditionally, the chest is opened through the breastbone to reach the heart. The patient is placed on a special heart-lung machine that continues to circulate oxygenated blood throughout the body when the heart is stopped during the surgery.

The surgeon then places the bypass grafts. If a vein is used, it's attached with very small stitches (sutures) to the aorta, the large artery leaving the heart with oxygenated blood. The vein is then attached to the coronary artery below the severe blockage. If the artery in the chest (called a mammary artery) is used, it is attached directly to the coronary artery below the blockage. This artery is already full of oxygenated blood.

When all the grafts are completed, the patient is removed from the heart-lung machine, and the heart is restarted. After this, the breastbone will be put back together with stainless steel wires.

Recovery takes place in an intensive care unit. After discharge from the hospital (which, depending on the patient, takes place three to five days after the surgery), post-operation recovery varies from person to person, but is usually six to eight weeks.

If bypass surgery is needed to treat CAD, the surgical team will supply detailed information regarding the risks and recovery. Today, new techniques using smaller incisions are being used. In certain situations, surgeons may opt to sew the bypasses into a beating heart, in which case the heart-lung-bypass machine is not needed. In this type of surgery, the recovery period is usually shortened.

Before ending this section, I need to reemphasize that in the acute treatment of CAD, the ultimate problem is severe blockages that prevent adequate blood flow in the artery. After the acute treatment is completed, these blockages must be addressed by preventive measures, which may help the blockages become smaller (regression) and more stable. Whether the arteries can be acutely treated successfully by angioplasty/stents or bypass surgery can be a difficult decision, with more than one "right" treatment available.

I haven't covered all the specific medications used for treatment of acute CAD here. In general, it is important for you to know that medications for CAD (1) lower and stabilize cholesterol levels, (2) lower the risk of clot formation, (3) increase blood flow to the heart, and (4) decrease the workload of the heart. The workload can be decreased by medications that slow the heart, lower the blood pressure, and dilate the arteries.

Chronic Coronary Artery Disease (CAD)

Because much of coronary artery disease is acquired, I want to focus on its treatment. To put it simply, we develop CAD largely because of daily decisions we make throughout a lifetime. Once we have CAD, we must look at our lifestyles and evaluate the choices we've made and are continuing to make.

Coronary artery disease—blockages in the arteries supplying blood to the heart—is the most common manifestation of a disease in the cardiovascular system. Much could be written about the chronic treatment, but I'll keep it short and, I hope, sweet.

We must lower cholesterol with good nutrition, sometimes used in concert with medications. When I say "good nutrition," I mean, ideally, a plant-based diet. We must also include daily exercise, maintain optimal body weight, keep blood pressure low, stay away from cigarettes and secondhand smoke, limit stress in our lives to the degree we have control over it, and laugh as much as is humanly possible. That's right. Laughter is good for the heart!

It's hard to admit that we contribute to the development of our own disease. But while genetics do play a role, much of disease is a result of the choices we make in taking care of those genes. Diet is a very personal subject. Our Westernized diet—high in fats and refined foods—contributes greatly to CAD. What foods are high in fat? Meat, eggs, cheese, and milk are major players in the development of CAD.

Also, the Western diet is high in sodium. What contains sodium? It's not so much the table salt that we sprinkle on for taste. It's the packaged, processed, canned foods that contain extremely high amounts of sodium and other chemicals that our bodies were not created to handle.

In parts of the world where a plant-based diet predominates, CAD is greatly reduced—sometimes even nonexistent. However, as the world has become more "Westernized," the disease rates in those same areas have skyrocketed. It only makes sense that the cornerstone of the treatment of chronic CAD must involve optimal nutrition.

Exercise does so many wonderful things for the body that it should definitely be considered a treatment. There are even times when exercise proves to be more effective than medications.

Daily exercise helps to lower the blood pressure, increases "good" cholesterol, lowers "bad" cholesterol, diminishes stress levels, helps prevent and treat diabetes, and keeps weight down. If all that weren't enough, exercise also keeps the inside lining of the blood vessels healthy. The list of benefits from exercise could go on and on, but I think you get the point that exercise is vital in treating chronic coronary artery disease.

Treating stress is also important in the management of chronic coronary artery disease. Chronic stress damages the body in many ways. It can cause development of bad coping mechanisms such as smoking, drinking alcohol, using drugs recreationally, and overeating. Stress hinders rest, raises blood pressure, and causes headaches and muscle pains throughout the body. Stress also increases the chance of experiencing a heart attack. Believe me, treating stress is crucial to the successful treatment of chronic coronary artery disease.

There are many other aspects, including getting appropriate rest and maintaining proper fluid consumption, but do not forget the big three—nutrition, exercise, and stress. Combating CAD demands a change in our chemical environment, which can be accomplished by the above methods. But how do we change a lifetime of bad habits and poor choices?

The power to do that doesn't lie in us. It can be found only in God. He gives us the power to make changes one at a time as we learn to depend on Him daily. This divine power is essential in not only the treatment of coronary disease but also in the achievement of our life goals. Studies have confirmed that patients with active spiritual lives do better in other areas of their personal lives.

As we gain the power to make changes, we begin to feel better. This enables more and more positive changes to take place. Our chemical makeup will shift as we eat better, exercise, and deal with stress. The disease becomes stabilized, and even—incredibly—regresses. Yes—chronic coronary artery disease can be reversed! And the treatment requires discipline, hard work, and power from God.

As patients make these changes, they tell me they feel better than they have ever felt in their lives. They wouldn't go back to their previous habits for any reason.

Remember, our habits and the way we live contribute greatly to the problem. Even though we can place a stent in an artery or bypass blocked areas, we must also look at the larger picture and deal with the long-term aspects of the problem. If we fail to do this, the problem will recur. Let me repeat that. *If we fail to deal with the long-term aspects of the problem, the problem will recur.*

Now that we have discussed the treatment for chronic blockages, the most common problem in the cardiovascular system, let's move on to other treatments of the cardiovascular system.

Malfunction of the Electrical System
When the electrical system malfunctions, the heart goes too slowly, too quickly, or irregularly. In all these cases, the heart does not generate adequate pressure to pump blood to the body.

Slow Heart Rhythms
The malfunction is diagnosed as I described earlier. For abnormally slow heart rhythms, if no outside sources are causing the problem (for example, medications), the cardiologist recommends a pacemaker. A *pacemaker* is a small metal device consisting of a battery, electrical circuits, a computerlike sensor, and leads. The battery is placed under the skin, usually in the left upper-chest area near the collarbone. The leads, thin wires attached to the pacemaker, are directed into the right side of the heart. At the tip of each lead are electrodes that sense the heart's

activity and send electrical impulses to the heart if needed. Pacemaker placement is done under local anesthetic (numbing medicine and a medication to relax).

Pacemakers help the heart beat sequentially by sending electrical charges that cause the muscle to contract when needed. The pacemaker contains sensors that can monitor the heart's activity. Based on what these sensors detect, the pacemaker may or may not send electrical impulses. These devices are now very small, about the size of a matchbox, and can last approximately six to eight years, depending on the situation. The function of the pacemaker is evaluated by phone monthly and at visits to the cardiologist at six-month intervals.

An external control system is used to make adjustments. I can't think of a more important device than a pacemaker to extend patients' lives. People with pacemakers can participate in sports and live active lives. Patients carry a pacemaker card at all times to help in the rare case of a malfunction.

Rapid Heart Rhythms

In other electrical abnormalities, the electrical impulses speed through the heart too *fast*. A variety of treatments are available. At times, avoiding stimulants like caffeine, cigarettes, or alcohol can successfully treat rapid rhythms and palpitations. Any type of stress to the body including pain, strong emotions, or illness can cause the body's own natural signals to make the heart skip and beat faster.

Many medications are available for the treatment of rapid heart rhythms. The type of fast heart rhythm detected and the patient's overall medical status will determine treatment. The health care provider should discuss the pros and cons of these medications with the patient.

An abnormally fast rhythm can be treated by *cardioversion—*

a jolt of electricity from an outside source used to reset the heart. During this process the patient is mildly sedated—unless the procedure must be done in an emergency situation. Two paddles, or electrode pads, are applied to the front of the chest or the back and pass an electrical current through the heart with the goal of returning the heart's rhythm to normal. Sometimes the chest feels sore afterward.

There are occasions when groups of cells in the upper part of the heart can produce a fast, abnormal heart rhythm. This can be thought of as a "short circuit" in the system. Electrophysiologic testing (described in appendix 2) can identify the cause of these fast rhythms. A specialized cardiologist, called an electrophysiologist, can identify where these abnormal rhythms are originating. These areas can then be destroyed permanently with the use of sound waves in a process termed *catheter ablation*.

In some individuals, abnormally fast heart rhythms begin in the bottom part of the heart. These are often life threatening. Devices called *implantable defibrillators* can be placed to help correct this problem. These are similar to pacemakers but are slightly larger and made of titanium. They sense the dangerous rhythms and fire electrical impulses to terminate the abnormal rhythm. The impulses, or "shocks," can be uncomfortable. Special instructions are given to patients with defibrillators. The defibrillator has various programs for dealing with abnormal rhythms. Former Vice President Cheney had a defibrillator implanted while he was still in office.

Heart Failure

When the heart cannot pump adequately to meet the body's needs, heart failure is said to occur. There can be many different causes of heart failure. The heart muscle may be weak because of blockages in the arteries; the heart may be unable to relax; the electrical system may malfunction; toxins such as alcohol, chemotherapy, and radiation may damage the muscle; or the valves may function inadequately. There are also a host of other causes, including, but not limited to, infections, thyroid disease, certain medications, and sometimes inherited disease.

Treatment focuses on correcting the underlying cause, if possible. In addition, many medications are available to help a weak heart. Some of these medications help by blocking the hormones a failing heart generates, because high levels of these hormones can damage the heart further. In addition, lifestyle changes are recommended, including monitoring fluid intake and avoiding salt. Too much fluid or salt can overload the heart. Usually providers will recommend an exercise program. Recently, special pacemaker devices, called biventricular pacemakers, have been used to help certain weak hearts. If these measures are unsuccessful in controlling symptoms, some patients may be eligible for heart transplants. This would be a last resort, as donors are scarce. Before providers consider a transplant, they follow strict health criteria, including the exclusion of other serious health problems.

Valvular Malfunction

If a heart valve malfunctions and symptoms develop, the valve needs to be replaced or repaired. The timing of surgery is crucial to long-term success. A valve should not be replaced or repaired too soon, because there are risks involved in open-heart surgery. Conversely, if one waits too long, the heart may be further weakened, which leads to a more difficult surgery and recovery. A cardiologist will advise patients regarding timing. Often medications can be used to treat milder valvular problems.

It's important to determine whether a valve can be repaired instead of being replaced. If surgery is needed, a cardiovascular surgeon, along with a cardiologist, will determine which of the numerous heart valves available, including both mechanical valves and tissue valves, is the best replacement valve for the patient. The pros and cons of each kind of valve should be discussed before surgery.

This appendix does not mention treatments for every malfunction of the heart, but there is constantly new research being done for the treatment of heart disease.

Lately, there's even been research and evaluation on a new artificial heart. A left ventricular assist device is now available, which can help a weak heart pump blood. Some surgeons are removing dead heart muscle to improve heart function. Researchers are injecting growth factors into the heart to grow new blood vessels. Some researchers are using lasers to make small holes in the heart to assist it in obtaining more blood. And new medications are being developed for the treatment of heart disease. In the future, we'll possibly be hearing more about gene therapy as a method of treatment.

Myths about Treatment of Cardiovascular Disease

1. Once I've had bypass surgery, I cannot have a heart attack. This is false. Your risk is still present, but because of increased flow from the grafts, a future heart attack tends to be smaller.

2. Medications can prevent a heart attack. Certain medications lower the risk, but they do not eliminate the risk altogether.

Medications

The following table lists the types of medications used and their effects on the heart.

THE ULTIMATE PRESCRIPTION

Medication Classes Used to Treat Heart Disease	
ACE Inhibitors (angiotensin converting enzyme inhibitors)	Block the production of natural substances that cause blood vessels to narrow, thus lowering blood pressure. Also used to treat heart failure; help the heart to heal after heart attacks.
Alpha blockers	Relax the muscle around arteries, lowering blood pressure.
Angiotensin II (receptor blockers)	Lower blood pressure by blocking receptors that are used to constrict blood vessels; may help patients with weak hearts.
Antiarrhythmics	Help control abnormal heart rhythms.
Aspirin	Inhibits blood clotting by interacting with platelet function. Used to treat CAD.
Beta blockers	Block receptors that result in a slowing heart rate. Used for hypertension, CAD, and CHF (congestive heart failure).
Blood thinners	Work in different ways. Help prevent the formation of blood clots. Used in many situations.
Calcium channel blockers	Relax blood vessels, and some can slow heart rates. Used in hypertension, CAD, and in some rhythm problems.
Cholesterol-lowering medications—statins, fibric acid, niacin, and binders	Decrease cholesterol levels. Used to treat CAD. Some of these medications have been shown to reduce the risk of heart attack.
Digitalis	Increases contractions of the heart; can slow heart rate. Used in CHF and some arrhythmias.
Diuretics	Lower blood volume by increasing the amount of sodium and water removed through the kidneys. Can also cause loss of potassium. Used for hypertension and CHF.

Fibrinolytics (clot dissolvers)	Break up blood clots; used in acute myocardial infarction (heart attacks). Most useful when given within a few hours of a heart attack.
Inotropes	Increase the pumping ability of the heart. Used in CHF.
Nitrates	Help the coronary arteries to dilate and lower pressures in the heart. Useful in CAD and CHF.
Platelet receptor inhibitors	Block the ability of platelets to stick together and form clots. Used in CAD. Help prevent clot formation around stents.

Medication Pearls

If your doctor prescribes medication, it's important for you to have a working understanding of the following:

- Know why you are taking each medication and what the medication looks like.
- Understand the directions for taking each medication.
- Get prescriptions refilled at least a week before you anticipate running out.
- Know which medications, if any, have caused you problems.
- Keep medication in original container in a cool place.
- Don't take medication in the dark.
- Don't stop taking a medication without talking to your doctor first.
- If you have surgery, dental work, or emergency treatment, tell your provider which medications you are taking.
- Don't double up on a medication without professional advice.
- Never share your medications with others.
- Get all prescriptions filled at one pharmacy; they will have a complete record.

QUESTIONS FOR FURTHER THOUGHT OR DISCUSSION

Introduction

1. Dr. Marcum says that we are so caught up in what tastes good, feels good, and seems good that we have lost sight of what really is good (pg. xii). Do you agree with his assessment? If so, in what ways do you get caught up in this mentality?
2. How has the media influenced your character, ideals, mind, or health?

Chapter 1

1. What is your reaction to Dr. Marcum's statement that the world believes modern medicine can fix anything?
2. How do you feel that modern medical technology as described on pages 6-7 affects how you think about your health? Do you agree that there is a downside to advancing technology? Why or why not?

Chapter 2

1. Where do you get your information about how to have a healthy lifestyle? Who sets the standard for health in your life?
2. Dr. Marcum writes that the concept of food as a stressor may be new to some people. How might food be a stressor?

Chapter 3

1. How do you think society would be different if we focused on creating products specifically and intentionally aimed at good health?
2. Dr. Marcum states that "we were created to live in a perfect, love-filled world" (pg. 24). Do you agree with this statement? Why or why not? If this is true, what effect do you think that has on our health?

Chapter 4

1. What stressors, hidden or not, are affecting your health? What are some steps you could take to change this?
2. Do you understand how we can be led into stress without even realizing it?

Chapter 5

1. Dr. Marcum talks about how medications are perceived to have healing powers. Why do you think this has become a common belief?
2. Do you see a connection between religious activities and your health? Why or why not?
3. In what ways could a relationship with Jesus Christ improve your health?

Chapter 6

1. Dr. Marcum says that stress occurs when we live contrary to the original plan (pgs. 47-48). Are there ways in which you are living contrary to the original plan? If so, how?
2. In what ways have you not trusted God before but could start trusting Him now?
3. How do you respond to the story of the physics professor's test (pgs. 50-53)? How does this story relate to your health?

4. In what ways are you on course with God's Health Plan? In what ways do you need to improve?

Chapter 7

1. Dr. Marcum asks the question "Are you living in a physical, mental, or spiritual 'black hole'?" (pg. 58). How would you answer this question?
2. Like the worried woman waiting for her family to get home (pg. 58), how has the light of God's love affected your life and/or your health?

Chapter 8

1. When was the last time you took a deep breath? What stress in your life keeps you from breathing well?
2. How often do you "dilute" God? What is the result?

Chapter 9

1. Does food advertising influence your nutrition? Why or why not?
2. How has eating healthful foods had a positive impact on your mental and spiritual well-being?
3. Dr. Marcum states that healthy thoughts, commonsense exercise, focused worship, and loving hearts are also parts of building and maintaining optimum health. How do these play a part in your health plan?
4. How can healthy habits turn into idols in your life?
5. Of Dr. Marcum's thirteen practical suggestions (pgs. 89-91), which do you struggle with the most? Why?

Chapter 10

1. What is your reaction to Dr. Marcum's statement that sunlight is a biblical prescription?

2. How much sleep do you require to feel rested? What keeps you from getting the adequate sleep you need?

Chapter 11

1. In what ways is music a part of your life?
2. Dr. Marcum mentions that God doesn't always use instruments or voices to bring about his purpose. What sounds bring healing or calm to your life?
3. When was the last time you sang praises to God? How did you feel during/after?

Chapter 12

1. Dr. Marcum states that God wanted Adam to experience a sense of ownership, responsibility, and love in naming every living creature. How does God want that for you?
2. What activities do you do that are good for your health?
3. In what ways do you invite God into your health/exercise plan?

Chapter 13

1. How often do you observe a day of rest? How could having a day of rest affect your health? Your faith?
2. What activities could you participate in to maintain God's seven-day cycle?
3. Dr. Marcum uses sports as an example of something that can be worshiped. What do you worship? How does this get in the way of your relationship with God?

Chapter 14

1. Of the eight deceptions Dr. Marcum describes (pgs. 143-149), which is hardest for you to believe? Why?
2. Do you see examples of what Dr. Marcum calls the "ripple effect" in your life? In your health?

Chapter 15

1. When you think about your overall health, whose message do you think you listen to more: God's or society's? Why?
2. What lies are you listening to that affect your health?
3. How is Dr. Marcum's statement that "choice is a product of love not dominion" evident in your life?

Chapter 16

1. How do you respond to the statement "Lies believed break the circle of love and trust. This leads to a spirit of fear, selfishness, and rebellion" (p. 163)?
2. Do you feel that you are running from the One True Healer? Why or why not?

Chapter 17

1. In what ways do you live your life in fear?
2. What things or people in your life do you love? How has this love affected your health?
3. How have you seen love to be a healing element in your life?

Chapter 18

1. What are some ways God has revealed His love for you personally?
2. Dr. Marcum states that "when we love others, when we make them laugh, when we help them along life's way, we are giving them a great prescription." How are you doing this for the people in your life?
3. Do you believe that serving others can change your chemistry and bring healing to the body?

ABOUT THE AUTHOR

Dr. James L. Marcum is a board-certified behavioral cardiologist with a thriving practice at the prestigious Chattanooga Heart Institute. *USA Today*'s Qforma database named him one of the nation's most influential physicians. He and Charles Mills cohost *Heartwise*, a call-in radio program that airs on more than 500 radio stations around the globe. In addition to hosting the *Bible Rx* and *Heart of Health* television programs, Dr. Marcum is an in-demand speaker who specializes in boldly treading on health care topics normally overlooked in the highly marketed and profitable field of health care. Married with two children, Dr. Marcum lives in Chattanooga, Tennessee, and enjoys music, sports, and outdoor activities.

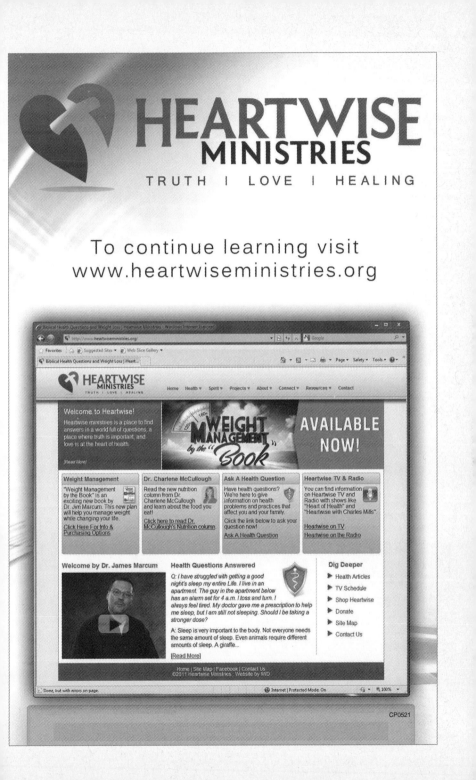